Centers for Disease Control and Prevention

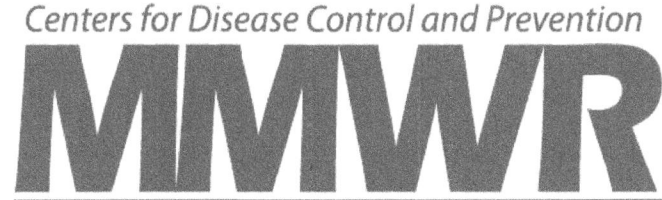

Morbidity and Mortality Weekly Report

Recommendations and Reports / Vol. 60 / No. 5

September 16, 2011

School Health Guidelines to Promote Healthy Eating and Physical Activity

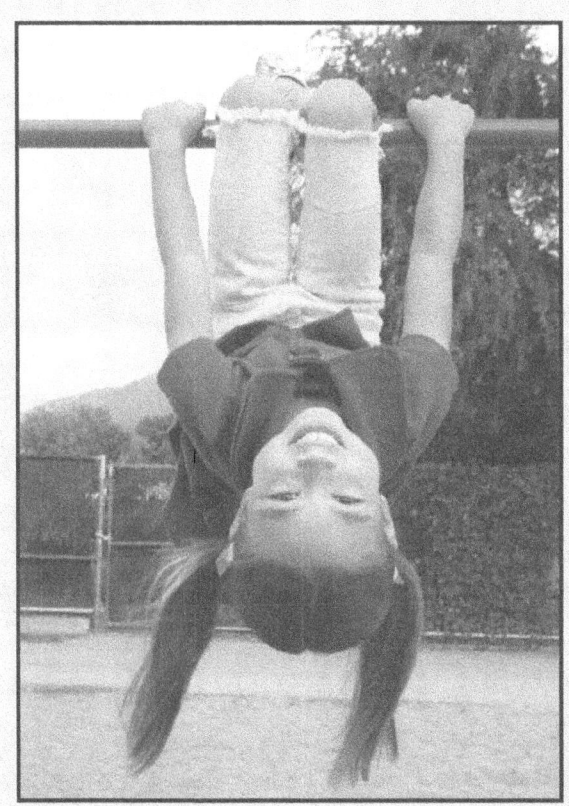

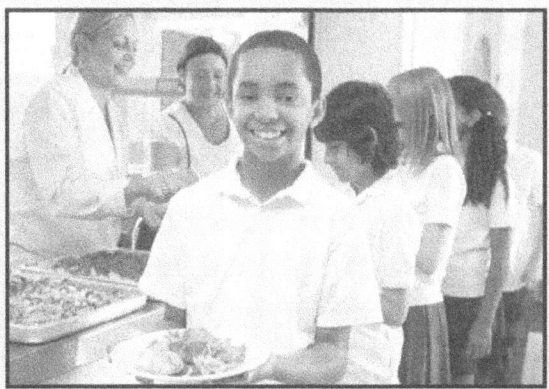

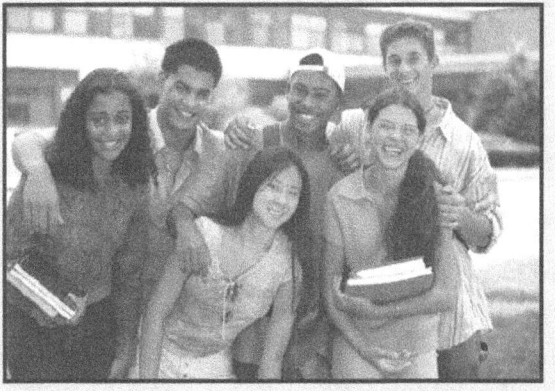

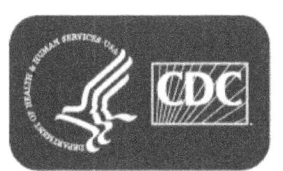

U.S. Department of Health and Human Services
Centers for Disease Control and Prevention

CONTENTS

CONTENTS (*Continued*)

The *MMWR* series of publications is published by the Office of Surveillance, Epidemiology, and Laboratory Services, Centers for Disease Control and Prevention (CDC), U.S. Department of Health and Human Services, Atlanta, GA 30333.

Suggested Citation: Centers for Disease Control and Prevention. [Title]. MMWR 2011;60(No. RR-#):[inclusive page numbers].

School Health Guidelines to Promote Healthy Eating and Physical Activity

Prepared by
Division of Adolescent and School Health,
National Center for Chronic Disease Prevention and Health Promotion

Summary

During the last 3 decades, the prevalence of obesity has tripled among persons aged 6–19 years. Multiple chronic disease risk factors, such as high blood pressure, high cholesterol levels, and high blood glucose levels are related to obesity. Schools have a responsibility to help prevent obesity and promote physical activity and healthy eating through policies, practices, and supportive environments.

This report describes school health guidelines for promoting healthy eating and physical activity, including coordination of school policies and practices; supportive environments; school nutrition services; physical education and physical activity programs; health education; health, mental health, and social services; family and community involvement; school employee wellness; and professional development for school staff members. These guidelines, developed in collaboration with specialists from universities and from national, federal, state, local, and voluntary agencies and organizations, are based on an in-depth review of research, theory, and best practices in healthy eating and physical activity promotion in school health, public health, and education. Because every guideline might not be appropriate or feasible for every school to implement, individual schools should determine which guidelines have the highest priority based on the needs of the school and available resources.

Background

Healthy eating and regular physical activity play a substantial role in preventing chronic diseases, including heart disease, cancer, and stroke, the three leading causes of death among adults aged >18 years (*1–5*). Poor diet and physical inactivity among younger persons can lead to an increased risk for certain chronic health conditions, including high blood pressure, type 2 diabetes, and obesity (*1*). During 2007–2008, 20% of U.S. children aged 6–11 years and 18% of persons aged 12–19 years were obese, percentages that have tripled since 1980 (*6*). Engaging children and adolescents in healthy eating and regular physical activity can lower their risk for obesity and related chronic diseases (*7,8*).

The dietary and physical activity behaviors of children and adolescents are influenced by many sectors of society, including families, communities, schools, child care settings, health-care providers, faith-based institutions, government agencies, the media, and the food and beverage industries and entertainment industry. Each of these sectors has an important, independent role to play in improving the dietary and physical activity behaviors of young persons. Schools play a particularly critical role by establishing a safe and supportive environment with policies and practices that support healthy behaviors. Schools also provide opportunities for students to learn about and practice healthy eating and physical activity behaviors.

Introduction

In response to the childhood obesity epidemic, much research has been conducted on school-based obesity prevention and healthy eating and physical activity promotion and intervention since the last publication of the *Guidelines for School and Community Programs to Promote Lifelong Physical Activity Among Young People* (1997) and the *Guidelines for School Health Programs to Promote Lifelong Healthy Eating* (1996). The new guidelines in this report synthesize the scientific evidence and best practices during 1995–2009 and combine healthy eating and physical activity into one set of evidence-based guidelines for schools serving students in kindergarten through 12th grade (grades K–12); other educational programs within schools, such as prekindergarten, might also be able to apply these guidelines in their settings. These guidelines support the 2010 *Dietary Guidelines for Americans* (*5*), the 2008 *Physical Activity Guidelines for Americans* (*9*), and the *Healthy People 2020* objectives related to healthy eating and physical activity among children and adolescents and schools (*10*). The guidelines establish a foundation for developing, implementing, and evaluating school-based healthy eating and physical

The material in this report originated in the National Center for Chronic Disease Prevention and Health Promotion, Ursula E. Bauer, PhD, Director
Corresponding preparer: Sarah M. Lee, PhD, CDC, National Center for Chronic Disease Prevention and Health Promotion, 4770 Buford Hwy NE, MS K-12, Atlanta, GA 30341. Telephone: 770-488-6126; Fax: 770-488-5771; E-mail: skeuplee@cdc.gov.

activity policies and practices for students (Appendix A). Each of the nine guidelines is accompanied by a series of strategies for schools to implement.

The primary audience for this report includes state and local education and health agencies, federal agencies, and national nongovernmental organizations that focus on the health of students in school. Agencies can use these guidelines to establish professional development materials, programs, and resources for partners and constituents. Locally, physical education and health education teachers, school nutrition directors, school health councils, and other school staff members; health-care providers; community members; policy makers; parents; and students can use these guidelines to establish, implement, and assess healthy eating and physical activity policies and practices in schools. Finally, faculty members in institutions of higher education can use these guidelines to teach students of school health, public health, physical education, health education, exercise and wellness, physical activity, dietetics, nutrition education, nursing, elementary and secondary education, and other health- and education-related disciplines.

Methods

This report updates and combines the previously published *Guidelines for School and Community Programs to Promote Lifelong Physical Activity Among Young People* (1997) and *Guidelines for School Health Programs to Promote Lifelong Healthy Eating* (1996) (*11,12*). The current guidelines and the corresponding strategies and actions were developed through a synthesis of scientific reports and expert opinion about effective and feasible practices in U.S. schools. Development of the guidelines involved an extensive literature search, development and use of a codebook by CDC staff members for rating the sufficiency of the scientific evidence and expert opinion, and an external review by approximately 50 organizations and persons in the fields of school health, education, public health, nutrition, and physical activity. (A list of these technical advisors is provided on page 76.) The use of practice-based expert opinion refines research-based guidelines to ensure that recommendations are accessible, given limited funding and resources; credible, allowing them to be implemented in various school settings and communities; and reasonable in terms of the expectations they set for professional practice and health outcomes (*13*).

Literature Search and Inclusion Criteria

CDC scientists conducted an extensive search for scientific reports, using five electronic citation databases: Medline, Cinahl, Sports Discus, PsychInfo, and ERIC. The coordinated school health approach was used to organize the literature search results for school-based nutrition and physical activity as they related to a healthy and safe school environment; nutrition services; physical education and school-based physical activity; health education; health services and counseling, psychological and social services; family and community involvement; and health promotion for staff members.

Scientific reports were included if they described practices to improve child and adolescent nutrition and physical activity that were based in schools or that addressed family or community involvement in schools. Two overall types of scientific reports were used to identify the new guidelines and corresponding strategies and actions: 1) reports that included cross-sectional, prospective, and randomized controlled trials that were designed to improve healthy eating and physical activity and prevent youth obesity and to promote wellness among school employees and 2) expert statements that included opinions, commentaries, or consensus statements from public health and education organizations or agencies about youth nutrition, physical activity, or obesity prevention. Scientific reports were included if they were published during 1995–2009 to update and expand on research described in the previous guidelines. Epidemiologic and surveillance data also were used to develop the introductory text.

Reports were excluded from consideration if they included only preschool children or college-age or older adults, were not in English, described clinical trials for weight-loss drugs or other nonbehavioral methods for weight loss, primarily addressed mental health issues such as eating disorders, or described interventions to improve performance in a specific sport or to improve functional ability after illness or injury.

A total of 6,213 abstracts were screened to identify full scientific reports to be retrieved. A total of 1,325 full scientific reports and expert statements were retrieved and reviewed for consideration in the guidelines.

Characteristics of Scientific Reports

A team of four CDC scientists used a database to record descriptions of each of the 1,325 scientific reports and expert statements, including health topics (e.g., nutrition, physical activity, and obesity prevention); component of the coordinated school health framework (e.g., physical education and health education); setting of the intervention (e.g., school, district, and community or county level); geographic location; age, sex, race/ethnicity, socioeconomic status, and health condition of participants; and topic of the report (e.g., policy and curricula). For reports describing evaluation studies, CDC scientists identified and documented the sample size, demographic makeup of study participants, duration of study, method of group assignment (e.g., random, quasiexperimental, or single group); length of follow-up after baseline measures; and outcomes of the study, such as impact on participant knowledge, attitude, behavior, or health status. Expert statements were described by type of statement (e.g., expert group statement, best practices document, or position statement), who convened the statement process, who funded the statement process, the nature of the convening group (e.g., established organization, ad hoc committee, federally sponsored committee, or CDC-funded grantee), and how evidence was presented in the expert statement.

Rating Sufficiency of Evidence

After describing the characteristics of evaluation studies and expert statements, four CDC staff members rated the relevance of each for inclusion in the guidelines. Each study and expert statement was read, and its evidence was rated. For scientific reports, the rating process focused on rigor, confidence in the findings, efficacy, and feasibility. For expert statements, the rating process focused on the organization that published or wrote the report, conflicts of interest, and evidence to support the statement.

Scientific Reports

Scientific reports were included if they had a rigorous study design with, at a minimum, a matched comparison group, strong study methods that contributed to confidence in the results, evaluation efficacy that included one or more positive results, and feasibility of implementing the intervention rated as medium or better. All four categories had to be rated as acceptable for a study to be included in the review for this guideline document.

In addition to the review of research and evaluation studies, CDC staff members identified, collected, and considered for inclusion all relevant reports from the Task Force on Community Preventive Services. Three task force reports on nutrition, physical activity, and obesity were relevant (i.e., applicable to school settings) and included recommendations from the task force.

Expert Statements

Best practice documents, position statements of individual persons or on behalf of organizations, and convened expert panels that covered topics related to youth physical activity and nutrition were included in the expert statements that were read and rated for sufficiency of evidence. Expert statements were included if 1) the experts had no conflicts of interest (i.e., financial support was reported and was provided by a federal agency or federal agency sponsor, a national nongovernmental organization such as the American Academy of Pediatrics, National Association for Sport and Physical Education, or American Dietetic Association, or a state-level health or education department); 2) the convening group was an established organization, federally sponsored committee, or a partner funded by the CDC Division of Adolescent and School Health; and 3) the expert statements could be associated with an evidence base (e.g., literature review and synthesis or meta-analysis).

Coding and Synthesis

To ensure standardized and reliable coding, four CDC staff worked in pairs to rate a subset of 40 reports. Discrepancies among coders were resolved through group discussion and consensus. The 1,325 scientific reports and expert statements were coded and categorized by each component for coordinated school health: healthy and safe school environment; nutrition services; physical education and school-based physical activity; health education; health services and counseling, psychological, and social services; family and community involvement; and school employee wellness. The CDC staff members concluded that there was enough scientific evidence on school-based nutrition and physical activity for each component of the coordinated school health framework to be an independent guideline. Furthermore, the CDC staff members identified enough scientific evidence to support the inclusion of two additional guidelines: 1) using a coordinated approach for nutrition and physical activity policies and practices and 2) professional development for school staff members. After identifying each guideline, the CDC staff members reviewed the scientific reports again to identify common strategies and actions within each guideline that resulted in positive associations with student knowledge, attitude, behavior, or health outcomes related to physical activity, diet, weight, or chronic disease risk factors. Expert statements also were reviewed for strategies and actions that are supported by opinions, commentaries, or consensus statements from public health and education organizations or agencies about youth nutrition, physical activity, or obesity prevention. Ultimately, 255 research and evaluation studies and 112 expert statements were rated as presenting evidence of sufficient relevance for a strategy or action to be included in the revision of the guidelines. An additional 343 descriptive articles were included in the document to support the background information (e.g., epidemiologic and surveillance data) included in the introduction and within each guideline.

Expert Input

In addition to the literature search and rating the sufficiency of the evidence, CDC convened a group of 10 experts in youth nutrition, physical activity, school health, school food service, education, and public health to review the scientific evidence and to provide individual input on proposed revisions of the guidelines. Input from the individual experts on the nine guidelines and corresponding strategies and actions were reviewed and integrated into the guidelines. CDC also garnered input from 53 federal and state education and public health agencies, as well as from nongovernmental organizations that represented policy makers, educators, parents, students, school nurses, physicians, and other health-care providers. Each of the 53 agencies provided a review of the guidelines and proposed revisions. The revised version was sent for review and revision to three experts in the field of school-based nutrition and physical activity who had not previously reviewed the document.

Epidemiologic Aspects of Healthy Eating and Physical Activity

Long-Term Outcomes of Healthy Eating and Physical Activity

This report was developed in response to the long-term and intermediate outcomes associated with inadequate physical activity and unhealthy eating. Healthy eating and physical activity have been associated with increased life expectancy, increased quality of life, and reduced risk for many chronic diseases (9,14–16). Healthy living through healthy eating and regular physical activity reduces the risk for the top three leading causes of death in the United States (heart disease, cancer, and stroke), as well as for certain chronic conditions, such as high blood pressure and type 2 diabetes (1,2,17).

Cardiovascular Disease

Cardiovascular disease (CVD) includes coronary heart disease, myocardial infarction, congestive heart failure, stroke, and other diseases and illnesses of the heart and blood vessels. Heart disease is the leading cause of death in the United States, and stroke is the third leading cause (18). Adult population subgroups disproportionately affected by CVD and its related risk factors include blacks, Hispanics, Mexican-Americans, and persons of low socioeconomic status (19). A healthy diet and regular physical activity can prevent and reduce metabolic risk factors that cause CVD, including hyperlipidemia (e.g., high cholesterol and triglyceride levels), high blood pressure, obesity, and insulin resistance and glucose intolerance (2,9,20). For example, dietary fiber can decrease the cholesterol concentration in the blood (21), and physical activity can help maintain normal blood glucose levels (9).

Studies indicate that CVD risk factors occur more frequently in obese children. Data from 2003–2006 National Health and Nutrition Examination Survey (NHANES) indicated that 3% of children and adolescents aged 8–17 years had increased blood pressure and that this risk was significantly greater among those who were obese (8%) (22). In a community-based sample of obese children aged 5–17 years, 70% had at least one CVD risk factor, such as a high cholesterol or triglyceride level, high blood pressure, or high insulin level, and 39% had two or more risk factors (23). However, among children of normal weight, 26% had at least one risk factor, and 13% had two or more risk factors (23).

Cancer

Cancer is the second leading cause of death in the United States, and black adults have a higher incidence rate of cancer than persons of any other racial/ethnic group (18,24). Some types of cancer can be prevented through regular physical activity and a diet consisting of various healthy foods with an emphasis on plant sources (e.g., fruits, vegetables, and whole grains) (17). A diet rich in plant foods is associated with a decreased risk for lung, esophageal, stomach, and colorectal cancer (17). Dietary factors that influence cancer risk include food type, variety, preparation, portion size, and fat content (17,25). Excess consumption of processed and red meats is associated with an increased risk for colorectal and prostate cancer (17).

Physical activity might contribute to cancer prevention through its role in regulating the production of hormones, boosting the immune system, and reducing insulin resistance (9). Regular physical activity can reduce the risk for developing cancers of the breast and colon, and some evidence indicates that physical activity can reduce the risk for developing endometrial and lung cancers (9). Healthy eating and physical activity also can contribute to cancer prevention by preventing obesity (9). Overweight and obesity are associated with increased risk for numerous types of cancer, including cancer of the breast, colon, endometrium, esophagus, kidney, pancreas, gall bladder, thyroid, ovary, cervix, and prostate, as well as multiple myeloma and Hodgkin's lymphoma (17).

Diabetes

Diabetes, a disease characterized by high blood glucose levels (26), was the seventh leading cause of death in the United States in 2007 (18). Diabetes is the leading cause of kidney failure, nontraumatic lower-extremity amputations, and new cases of blindness among adults and can affect the nervous system and oral health (26). Persons with diabetes have a two to four times higher risk for dying from CVD than those without diabetes (27,28). Diabetes is a result of defects in insulin production, insulin action, or both and is classified as either type 1 (insulin-dependent diabetes) or type

2 (usually non–insulin-dependent diabetes) (26). Although diet and physical activity can help control blood glucose levels and reduce complications from both types of diabetes, type 1 diabetes is an autoimmune disease of the pancreas, and little is known about prevention (29). In 2001, the prevalence of type 1 diabetes among a sample of U.S. persons aged 10–19 years was 2.28 cases per 1,000 persons (30).

Type 2 diabetes is the most common form of diabetes in adults (26). Healthy eating and regular physical activity can help prevent this type of diabetes (29,31,32). Type 2 diabetes was previously observed primarily among adults but has become more common among children and adolescents (26,29). In 2001, the prevalence of type 2 diabetes in a sample of U.S. persons aged 10–19 years was 0.42 cases per 1,000 persons (30) and was greatest among Asian/Pacific Islander, black, Hispanic, and American Indian persons (33). In the Pima Indian community, type 2 diabetes in children and adolescents aged 5–14 years increased significantly from 0.5 cases per 1,000 person-years in 1965–1977 to 3.3 cases per 1,000 person-years in 1991–2003 (32). According to the 2005–2006 NHANES, 16% (overall) of persons aged 12–19 years and 30% of obese persons aged 12–19 years had prediabetes, a condition in which blood glucose levels indicate a high risk for development of diabetes (26,34).

Intermediate Outcomes of Healthy Eating and Physical Activity

Poor diet and physical inactivity are risk factors for numerous conditions that affect overall health and quality of life, and many of these conditions can lead to chronic diseases. Intermediate outcomes such as obesity, metabolic syndrome, inadequate bone health, undernutrition, iron deficiency, eating disorders, and dental caries can begin in childhood, leading to earlier onset of disease and subsequent premature death.

Obesity

Healthy eating and physical activity control body weight through a balance of energy expenditure and caloric consumption (35). Weight gain occurs when persons expend less energy through physical activity than they consume through their diet (35). As this imbalance continues over time, the risk for overweight and obesity increases (35). Overweight is defined as having excess body weight for a particular height from fat, muscle, bone, water, or a combination of these factors (36). Obesity is the condition of excess body fat (37). Body mass index (BMI) is a ratio of weight and height (kilograms/meters^2) and is the most widely used and recommended measure to estimate weight status. In adults, weight status is determined directly by BMI. Among adults aged ≥20 years, overweight is classified as BMI ≥25 to <30 kg/m^2; obesity is classified as BMI ≥30 kg/m^2. Weight status in persons aged 2–19 years is determined by comparing their BMI to other persons of the same sex and age in a reference population. BMI is calculated and plotted by age on a sex-specific growth chart to determine a BMI-for-age percentile. Among persons aged 2–20 years, overweight is classified as BMI ≥85th to <95 percentile for age and sex; obesity is classified as BMI ≥95th percentile for age and sex (38).

In 2008, the prevalence of obesity among children aged 6–11 years was 20%, nearly triple the prevalence in 1980 (7%) (6,39–41). The rate among persons aged 12–19 years more than tripled over the same period, increasing from 5% to 18% (6,39–41). A Healthy People 2020 national health objective (nutrition and weight status [NWS]) is to reduce the proportion of children aged 6–11 years who are obese to 16% and reduce the proportion of persons aged 12–19 years who are obese to 16% by 2020 (objectives NWS 10.2 and NWS 10.3).

Since 1980, blacks aged <20 years have experienced greater BMI increases than both white and Mexican-American persons of the same age (42). During 2007–2008, non-Hispanic black females aged 2–19 years had significantly higher odds of being obese (23%) compared with non-Hispanic white females (15%); Hispanic males aged 2–19 years had significantly higher odds of being obese (24%) compared with non-Hispanic white males (16%) (6). Other evidence suggests that childhood obesity is significantly more common in American Indian/ Alaska Native children than in white or Asian children (43). In addition, a greater percentage of adolescents from families in poverty are obese (23%) compared with those from families not in poverty (14%) (44). (Poverty is determined by the poverty-income ratio, which is the ratio of a family's income to the U.S. Census Bureau's poverty threshold. The threshold varies with the number and ages of family members and is revised yearly.)

Obesity in children and adolescents is associated with numerous immediate health risks, including high blood pressure, high blood cholesterol levels, type 2 diabetes, metabolic syndrome, sleep disturbances, orthopedic problems, and social and psychological problems, such as discrimination and poor self-esteem (7,35,45). These immediate health risks can have long-term consequences for children and adolescents, affecting them into adulthood. Insufficient public health and education efforts to decrease or minimize these health risks will affect both health-care and education systems.

Increasing rates of obesity among children and adolescents are of particular concern because those who are obese are more likely to become overweight or obese adults and have related chronic diseases (8). The probability of childhood obesity persisting into adulthood increases as children enter adolescence

(46,47); even obesity during early childhood (ages 2–5 years) increases the risk for adult obesity (47–49). For example, a community-based study found that among boys aged 9–11 years, 4% of those with a childhood BMI <50th percentile (normal weight) and 22% of those with a childhood BMI of 50th–84th percentile (normal weight) became obese adults, whereas 76% of those who were obese (BMI ≥95th percentile) became obese adults. The findings were consistent for both sexes and all childhood age groups studied in the cohort (2–5 years, 6–8 years, 9–11 years, 12–14 years, 15–17 years) (47). Obesity in adults is associated with an increased risk for premature death, heart disease, type 2 diabetes, stroke, several types of cancer, osteoarthritis, and many other health problems (8,50). The risk factors and precursors to these diseases are being detected in obese children (23), and national concern exists that this trend might lower the age of onset of chronic conditions and diseases and possibly decrease the quality of life or shorten the lifespan of obese children (51).

Metabolic Syndrome

Metabolic syndrome is a clustering of metabolic risk factors that increases the risk for prematurely developing CVD and type 2 diabetes (52). Metabolic syndrome is defined as the presence of three or more of the following metabolic risk factors: abdominal obesity, high triglyceride levels, low high-density lipoprotein cholesterol (HDL-C) levels, high blood pressure, and high fasting glucose levels (52). Physical inactivity and obesity are established risk factors for metabolic syndrome, and a poor diet can accelerate the risk for developing CVD among persons with metabolic syndrome (52). A total of 27% of U.S. adults in 2004 (53) and 9% of adolescents in 2010 had metabolic syndrome (54), with Hispanic males having the highest prevalence among adolescents (54). In 2003, metabolic syndrome was significantly more prevalent among obese persons than among those of normal weight (55).

Inadequate Bone Health

According to the 2004 Surgeon General's report on bone health and osteoporosis, diet and physical activity are responsible for 10%–50% of bone mass and structure (56). Adequate calcium and vitamin D intake, along with weight-bearing physical activity (e.g., walking, jogging, and weightlifting), provide bones with proper support for healthy growth. Physical activity places a mechanical load on the skeleton, and the body responds by strengthening bone mass to support the activity. In addition, both vitamin D and regular physical activity enhance the positive effects of calcium (56).

Bone growth during adolescence is particularly crucial for achieving optimal bone health because bone mass peaks in late adolescence (56,57). Adolescents who do not achieve optimal bone mass during this period will lack the adequate support to sustain normal losses of bone mass later in life. Low body weight, weight loss, physical inactivity, and dieting among children and adolescents can lead to low bone density. Low bone density leads to osteoporosis, which is the most common cause of fractures among adults. In older adults, fractures lead to physical disabilities, depression, reduced quality of life, and potentially death (56,57). In 2004, approximately 10 million U.S. adults aged >50 years had osteoporosis, and an additional 33 million U.S. adults had the precursor condition, osteopenia (low bone mass). These conditions disproportionately affect women (56). In addition, obesity in children and adolescents is associated with orthopedic complications such as fractures, musculoskeletal pain, impairment in mobility, and abnormal lower extremity alignment (58).

Food Insecurity

Reduced food intake and disrupted eating patterns because a household lacks money and other resources for food is referred to as food insecurity. In 2008, approximately 49.1 million persons in the United States lived in food-insecure households, including 16.7 million children and adolescents, or 23% of all U.S. children and adolescents (59). Blacks and Hispanics have the highest prevalence of undernutrition (60), and food insecurity and hunger might be associated with lower dietary quality and undernutrition in children and adolescents, especially in adolescents (61). Undernutrition can have lasting effects on overall health, cognitive development, and school performance (62–65). Children and adolescents in food-insecure households have poorer health status and experience more frequent stomachaches and headaches than those from food-secure households (62). In addition to poor health outcomes, behavioral and psychosocial problems also have been associated with food insecurity and hunger in children and adolescents (62–64,66). Those who are food insecure have lower physical functioning and quality of life (67).

Children and adolescents experiencing hunger have lower math scores and are more likely to repeat a grade in school and receive special education services or mental health counseling than those not experiencing hunger (62,63). Children and adolescents experiencing hunger also are more likely to be absent and tardy from school than other children and adolescents (64). Schools have a long history of seeking out and developing strategies to address these concerns. The National School Lunch Program and School Breakfast Program were initiated, in part, as a way to reduce undernutrition among children and adolescents (68).

Iron Deficiency

Iron deficiency is a condition resulting from too little iron in the body (69). Iron deficiency hampers the body's ability to produce hemoglobin, which is needed to carry oxygen in the blood. This deficiency can increase fatigue, shorten attention span, decrease work capacity, impair psychomotor development, affect physical activity, and reduce resistance to infection (70,71). Iron deficiency ranges from depleted iron stores without functional or health impairment to iron deficiency with anemia, which affects the functioning of several body systems (70). To prevent iron deficiency, children and adolescents need to consume adequate amounts of foods containing iron (e.g., meat, poultry, egg yolk, dried fruit, dried peas and beans, nuts, green leafy vegetables, whole grain breads, and fortified cereals), as well as foods high in vitamin C (e.g., citrus fruits, tomatoes, melons, peppers, greens, cabbage, broccoli, strawberries, kiwis, and potatoes), to help the body absorb iron efficiently (70). Among school-age children and adolescents with iron deficiency, anemia is associated with poor cognition and lower academic performance (72,73). Whether this association exists among iron-deficient children and adolescents without anemia is unclear (73).

A *Healthy People 2020* national health objective strives to reduce iron deficiency among young children (aged 1–4 years) and females of childbearing age (aged 12–49 years) (objective NWS 21) (10). Among females aged 12–19 years, the prevalence of iron deficiency is 9% (74). In a national sample, children and adolescents who were overweight or obese were approximately twice as likely to be iron deficient than those of normal weight (75).

Eating Disorders

Eating disorders are psychological disorders characterized by severe disturbances in eating behavior. Anorexia nervosa is characterized by a refusal to maintain a normal body weight. Bulimia nervosa is characterized by repeated episodes of binge eating followed by compensatory behaviors such as self-induced vomiting (76). Disorders that do not meet all criteria for either anorexia nervosa or bulimia nervosa are referred to as eating disorders not otherwise specified.

Eating disorders are more common in females than males. Among females, the lifetime prevalence of anorexia nervosa is approximately 0.5%, and the lifetime prevalence of bulimia nervosa is 1%–3% (76). The prevalence of anorexia nervosa and bulimia nervosa in males is approximately one tenth that in females.

According to the American Psychiatric Association, the prevalence of anorexia nervosa and bulimia nervosa in U.S. children and younger adolescents is not well documented (77). However, children and adolescents report disordered eating behaviors that are clinically severe but do not meet full criteria for an eating disorder. For example, in 2009, in a nationally representative sample of high school students, 11% of students had gone without eating for >24 hours; 5% had taken diet pills, powders, or liquids without a physician's advice; and 4% had vomited or taken laxatives to lose weight or to keep from gaining weight during the 30 days before the survey (78). Eating disorders can cause severe complications, and mortality rates for these disorders are among the highest for any psychiatric disorder (79).

Dental Caries

Dental caries is the most common chronic condition in children and adolescents, with the greatest prevalence in blacks and Mexican-Americans and in those who live in poverty (80). Pain from untreated caries can affect school attendance, eating, speaking, and subsequent growth and development (80). Dental caries is associated with sugar and full-calorie soda consumption (80,81). Children who are obese have been found to have higher rates of dental caries than their normal weight peers (82).

Healthy Eating Recommendations

The *Dietary Guidelines for Americans* have been published every 5 years since 1980 (5). These guidelines provide authoritative advice for persons aged ≥2 years on establishing dietary habits that promote health and reduce the risk for chronic disease. The guidelines recommend a diet rich in fruits and vegetables, whole grains, and fat-free and low-fat dairy products for persons aged ≥2 years. The guidelines also recommend that children, adolescents, and adults limit intake of solid fats (major sources of saturated and trans fatty acids), cholesterol, sodium, added sugars, and refined grains (5). National health objectives include increasing the consumption of fruits, vegetables, whole grains, and calcium among persons aged ≥2 years, reducing consumption of calories from solid fats and added sugars, reducing consumption of saturated fats, and reducing sodium consumption (objectives NWS-14 through NWS-21) (10).

Eating Behaviors of Children and Adolescents

Available data indicate that most children and adolescents do not follow critical dietary guidelines. For example, the 2010 guidelines provide guidance on the amount of fruits and vegetables that children and adolescents should consume. The recommendation for persons aged 5–18 years is 2½–6½ cups of fruits and vegetables each day, depending on age and calorie requirements (5). However, most U.S. children and adolescents do not follow the recommendations for the numbers of daily servings or variety consumed (*3*). Furthermore, according to the 2009 national Youth Risk Behavior Survey (YRBS), only 22% of students in grades 9–12 reported consuming fruits and vegetables five or more times per day (*78*). The guidelines also recommend that children aged 4–8 years drink 2 cups of fat-free or low-fat milk or equivalent milk products per day and persons aged 9–18 years drink 3 cups per day (i.e., 1,300 mg/day), yet most children and adolescents do not drink the recommended amounts (*3*). A total of 15% of students in grades 9–12 drank three or more glasses of milk per day in 2009 (*5,78*). During 2007–2008, females aged 12–19 years had a particularly low intake of calcium, consuming an average of 878 mg of calcium daily, which is 67% of the recommended dietary allowance (*5,83*). In addition, from the 1970s through the mid-1990s, milk consumption among female adolescents decreased 36% (*84*).

The guidelines recommend that children and adolescents consume at least half of their daily grain intake as whole grains, which for many people is 2- to 3-oz equivalents, depending on age, sex, and calorie level (*5*). Whole grains are an important source of fiber and other nutrients. Persons aged 4–18 years do not eat the minimum recommended amounts of whole grains. During 2001–2004, the median intakes of whole grains in this age group ranged from 0.26–0.48 oz, far less than the recommended amounts (*3*).

During 2007–2008, the average percentage of calories from fat consumed by persons aged 6–19 years was 33%. Although these percentages are similar to those suggested by the dietary guidelines for total fat consumption (25%–35% of total calories), persons aged 6–19 years consumed more than the recommended amount of saturated fat (10% of total calories), ranging from 11%–12% (*5,83*).

Sodium intake, which is associated with increased blood pressure (*85*), has increased steadily during the last 35 years, in large part because of increased consumption of processed foods such as salty snacks and increased frequency of eating food away from home (*84*). The guidelines recommend a maximum daily intake of sodium of 2,300 mg or 1,500 mg, depending on age and other individual characteristics. African Americans; persons with hypertension, diabetes, or chronic kidney disease; and persons aged ≥51 years should have a sodium consumption of <1,500 mg/day. These groups make up approximately half of the U.S. population aged ≥2 years. However, almost all persons in the United States consume more than the recommended amount of sodium. During 2007–2008, boys aged 6–11 years and 12–19 years had an average daily sodium intake of 3,169 mg and 3,990 mg, respectively. Girls aged 6–11 and 12–19 years had an average daily sodium intake of 2,717 mg and 3,013 mg, respectively (*83*).

Although the dietary guidelines do not have a recommendation for the maximum daily intake for added sugar, they do recommend that persons reduce their intake of added sugars (*5*). Children and adolescents tend to have diets high in added sugar (*84*), with added sugar contributing approximately 18% of their total daily calories (*86*). Sugar-sweetened beverages (such as soda and fruit drinks) are major contributors to added sugar consumption and contribute an average of 8% of energy intake among persons aged 2–18 years (*86*). Males aged 12–19 years consume an average of 22.0 oz of full-calorie soda per day, more than twice their intake of fluid milk (9.8 oz); females consume an average of 14.3 oz of full-calorie soda and 6.3 oz of fluid milk (*87*). Because many foods and beverages with added sugar tend to contain few or no essential nutrients or dietary fiber, the guidelines advise that one way to reduce intake of added sugar is to replace sweetened foods and beverages with those that are free of or low in added sugars (*5*). In addition, empty calories from added sugar and solid fats contribute 40% of daily calories for persons aged 2–18 years, affecting overall diet quality (*86*). Approximately half of these empty calories come from six sources, which include soda, fruit drinks, dairy desserts, grain desserts, pizza, and whole milk (*86*).

The guidelines recommend that persons in the United States, including children and adolescents, strive to achieve and maintain a healthy body weight. Specifically, children and adolescents are encouraged to maintain the calorie balance needed to support normal growth and development without promoting excess weight gain (*5*). During 1971–2000, a significant increase in caloric intake occurred in the United States (*88*). Changes in energy intake among children and adolescents varied by age. Studies indicate that the overall energy intake among children (aged 2–5 and 6–11 years) remained relatively stable from 1971 to the late 1990s and 2000 (*84,89,90*). However, the energy intake among persons aged 12–19 years increased significantly during the same period (*84,90,91*).

Factors that Influence the Eating Behaviors of Children and Adolescents

Multiple factors, including demographic, personal, and environmental factors, influence the eating behaviors of children and adolescents. Male adolescents report greater consumption of fruits and vegetables and higher daily intakes of calcium, dairy servings, and milk servings than females (*78,92*). Black adolescents are more likely than white or Hispanic adolescents to report eating fruits and vegetables five or more times per day (*78*). Children and adolescents from low-income households are less likely to eat whole grain foods (*93*).

Taste preferences of children and adolescents are a strong predictor of their food intake (*94*). Taste preference for milk, among both males and females, is associated with calcium intake (*92*). Taste preferences for fruits and vegetables are one of the strongest reported correlates of fruit and vegetable intake among males and females (*94*). Male and female adolescents who reported frequent fast-food restaurant visits (three or more visits in the past week) were more likely to report that healthy foods tasted bad, that they did not have time to eat healthy foods, and that they cared little about healthy eating (*95*).

Certain behaviors and attitudes among children and adolescents are related to healthy eating. For example, behavior-change strategies that are initiated by children and adolescents (e.g., setting goals for fruit and vegetable intake or rewarding themselves for eating fruits and vegetables) and positive feelings toward eating fruits and vegetables are predictors of fruit and vegetable intake (*95*). Among female adolescents, self-efficacy to make healthy food choices and positive attitudes toward nutrition and health are significantly related to calcium intake (*92*).

The home environment and parental influence are strongly correlated with youth eating behaviors. Home availability of healthy foods is one of the strongest correlates of fruit, vegetable, and calcium and dairy intakes (*92,94*). Family meal patterns, healthy household eating rules, and healthy lifestyles of parents influence fruit, vegetable, calcium and dairy, and dietary fat intake of adolescents (*94–97*).

The physical food environment in the community, including the presence of fast-food restaurants, grocery stores, schools, and convenience stores, influences access to and availability of foods and beverages (*98*). A lack of grocery stores in neighborhoods is associated with reduced access to fresh fruits and vegetables (*99,100*) and less healthy food intake (*101*). Low-income neighborhoods have fewer grocery stores than middle-income neighborhoods, predominantly black neighborhoods have half the number of grocery stores as predominantly white neighborhoods, and predominantly Hispanic neighborhoods have one third the amount of grocery stores as predominantly non-Hispanic neighborhoods (*102*). Furthermore, lower-income and minority neighborhoods tend to have more fast-food restaurants than high-income and predominately white neighborhoods (*101*)

During 1994–1998, approximately three in 10 children and adolescents consumed at least one fast-food meal per day; those who reported eating fast foods consumed more total calories than those who did not (*103*). Children and adolescents who report eating fast foods tend to consume more total energy, fat, and sugar-sweetened beverages and consume less milk, fruits, and nonstarchy vegetables (*103*). Children and adolescents are more likely than adults to report fast-food consumption (*104*).

The school environment also influences youth eating behaviors and provides them with opportunities to consume an array of foods and beverages throughout the school day.

The widespread availability of foods and beverages served outside of the federal school lunch and breakfast programs is well-documented (*105,106*). These products, referred to as competitive foods and beverages because they are sold in competition with traditional school meals, often are sold in the school cafeteria and are available throughout school buildings, on school grounds, or at school-sponsored events. Results from a nationally representative survey found that in the 2004–2005 school year, one or more sources of competitive foods were available in 75% of elementary schools, 97% of middle schools, and 100% of high schools (*106*).

Food advertising and marketing influence food and beverage preferences and purchase requests of children and adolescents (i.e., when a child asks a parent to buy a specific item) and influence the dietary intake of children and adolescents (*107*). Children and adolescents are exposed to many forms of marketing, including television advertisements, advertising on the Internet and advergames (i.e., interactive, electronic games on a company-sponsored website that prominently feature one or more of the company's products or services), contests and prizes, television and movie product placement, marketing in schools (e.g., school score boards, vending machines, book covers, and homework incentives), and use of licensed characters to promote foods or restaurants. In a recent report to Congress, the Federal Trade Commission estimated that in 2006, approximately $1.6 billion was spent promoting foods, beverages, and fast-food restaurants to children (*108*). Because of the concern regarding the effect of food marketing on the diets of children and adolescents, Congress ordered the creation of an Interagency Working Group on Food Marketing to Children in 2009 to develop recommendations for foods marketed to persons aged <18 years.

Physical Activity Recommendations

Physical activity is defined as "any bodily movement produced by the contraction of skeletal muscle that increases energy expenditure above a basal level" (*9*). Examples of physical activity include walking, running, bicycling, swimming, jumping rope, active games, resistance exercises, and household chores. In the 2008 *Physical Activity Guidelines for Americans,* the U.S. Department of Health and Human Services (HHS) recommends that children and adolescents engage in ≥60 minutes of physical activity daily. Most of the ≥60 minutes/day should be either moderate- or vigorous-intensity aerobic physical activity. The guidelines indicate that children and adolescents should include vigorous intensity, muscle-strengthening, and bone-strengthening activities at least 3 days of the week. HHS also recommends encouraging children and adolescents to participate in activities that are age appropriate, are enjoyable, and offer variety (*9*). *Healthy People 2020* national health objectives include an objective on increasing the proportion of adolescents who meet current federal physical activity (PA) guidelines for aerobic physical activity and for muscle-strengthening activity (objective PA 3) (*10*).

Physical Activity Behaviors of Children and Adolescents

Despite national guidelines for physical activity, many young persons are not regularly physically active. In 2002, 62% of children and adolescents aged 9–13 years did not participate in any organized physical activity during nonschool hours, and 23% did not engage in any free-time physical activity (*109*). The 2009 national YRBS indicated that only 18% of high school students had been physically active for 60 minutes every day in the previous week (*78*). In 2009, although 56% of high school students reported being enrolled in physical education, only 33% of high school students nationwide attended physical education classes 5 days in an average school week, a decrease from 1991, when 43% of students attended physical education classes 5 days/week (*78*). Nationwide, 58% of high school students reported playing on at least one sports team run by their school or a community group in 2009 (*78*). As of 2005, <15% of children and adolescents walked or bicycled to and from school (*110*).

Factors that Influence the Physical Activity of Children and Adolescents

Regular participation in physical activity among children and adolescents is related to demographic, personal, social, and environmental factors. Hispanic and non-Hispanic black students are less active than their non-Hispanic white counterparts (*78*). In 2009, 20% of non-Hispanic white high school students, compared with 16% of Hispanic students and 17% of non-Hispanic black students, had been physically active for 60 minutes every day in the previous week (*78*). This difference also is evident during childhood and continues through adulthood, with non-Hispanic white adults having the highest prevalence of activity compared with other ethnic groups (*111*).

Sex is correlated with physical activity levels, with males participating in more overall physical activity than females (*112–118*). The 2009 national YRBS indicated that 25% of males and 11% of females had been physically active doing any kind of physical activity for at least 60 minutes per day in the previous week (*78*). This trend continues through adulthood, with females remaining less physically active than males (*119*). Adolescent males also report a greater intention to be physically active in the future than females (*120*).

Children and adolescents who intend to be active in the future and who believe physical activity is important for a healthy lifestyle engage in more activity. Overall, personal fulfillment influences the motivation both of boys and girls to be physically active (*121*). Child and adolescent perceptions of their ability to perform a physical activity (i.e., self-efficacy) and perceived competence affects their participation in the activity (*112,121–123*). Girls are motivated by physical activities that they prefer and by their confidence in their ability to perform an activity (*123*). Boys are affected by their ability to perform a particular physical activity, as well as by social norms among both friends and parents (*123*).

Positive social norms and support from friends and family encourage youth involvement in physical activity among all children and adolescents (*112,122,124–132*). Parent and family support for physical activity can be defined as a child's perception of support (e.g., perceiving parents will do physical activity with them and sign them up for sports or other physical activities) to a parent's reported support (e.g., regular encouragement of physical activity or regularly placing value on being active). Youth perceptions and parent reports of support for physical activity are strongly associated with participation in both structured and nonstructured physical activity among children and adolescents (*112,122,133–135*).

The physical environment can be both a benefit and a barrier to being physically active. Environmental factors that might pose a barrier to physical activity include low availability of safe locations to be active, perceived lack of access to physical activity equipment, cost of physical activities, and time constraints (*126,136–138*). Youth perceptions of neighborhood safety (e.g., traffic, strangers, poorly maintained or unsafe facilities, poor lighting, or negative social influences) also are associated with physical activity participation (*139–142*). Parents' perceptions about environmental factors also influence physical activity among children and adolescents. For example, parents rate distance and safety as top barriers for their children walking to school (*143*).

The school environment can also influence the participation of children and adolescents in physical activity. In 2006, 4% of elementary schools, 8% of middle schools, and 2% of high schools provided daily physical education for the entire school year for students in all grades in the school (*144*). Although this is a critical opportunity for children and adolescents to participate in physical activity, schools do not provide it daily. In addition, many schools do not regularly provide other physical activity opportunities during the school day, such as recess. In 2006, 26% of elementary schools did not provide regularly scheduled recess for students in all grades in the school (*144*). When schools provide supportive environments by enhancing physical education (*145,146*) and health education (*147*), having staff members become role models for physical activity, increasing communication about the benefits of physical activity, and engaging families and communities in physical activity, children and adolescents are more likely to be physically active and maintain a physically active lifestyle (*147–149*).

Television Viewing and Other Screen-Based Media Behaviors of Children and Adolescents

Television viewing, nonactive computer use, and nonactive video and DVD viewing are all considered sedentary behaviors. Television viewing among children and adolescents, in particular, has been shown to be associated with childhood and adult obesity (*150–157*). Potential mechanisms through which television viewing might lead to childhood obesity include 1) lower resting energy expenditure, 2) displacement of physical activity, 3) food advertising that influences greater energy intake, and 4) excess eating while viewing (*158,159*).

The American Academy of Pediatrics (AAP) recommends no more than 2 hours of quality television and video viewing (e.g., educational television programs) per day for children aged ≥2 years (*160*). Overall, persons aged 8–18 years spend an average of 7 hours and 11 minutes per day watching television, using a computer, and playing video games (*161*). In 2009, 33% of 9th- through 12th-grade students reported watching ≥3 hours of television on an average school day, and 25% reported using a computer ≥3 hours on an average school day (*78*). Black high school students most frequently reported excessive television viewing (≥3 hours/day) (56%), compared with their Hispanic (42%) and non-Hispanic white (25%) counterparts. Non-Hispanic black and Hispanic students also were more likely to report excessive computer use (≥3 hours/day) (30% and 26%, respectively) compared with non-Hispanic white students (22%) (*78*).

The home environment offers children and adolescents many opportunities for television viewing, including eating meals while watching television or having a television in their bedroom (*162–165*). The presence of a television in a child's bedroom is associated with more hours spent watching television (0.25 hours/day) (*163*), more time engaged in video games (0.31 hours/day), more time using computers (0.21 hours/day) (*163*), and obesity (*162,164,166,167*). The likelihood of having a television in the bedroom increases with a child's age (*163,167*).

Eating meals in front of the television is associated with more viewing hours (*163*). Children and adolescents are more likely to engage in unhealthy eating behaviors when watching television (*155,168,169*) and are exposed to television advertisements promoting primarily restaurants and unhealthy food products (*151,170*). Increased television viewing among children and adolescents is associated with consuming more products such as fast food, soft drinks, and high-fat snacks (*151,156,165,171–173*) and consuming fewer fruits and vegetables (*151,155,174*).

Healthy People 2020 Objectives for Healthy Eating and Physical Activity Among Children and Adolescents

Healthy People 2020 national health objectives include a comprehensive plan for health promotion and disease prevention in the United States. *Healthy People 2020* includes objectives related to physical activity and healthy eating among children and adolescents and in schools (Appendix B) (*10*).

Rationale for School Health Programs to Promote Healthy Eating and Physical Activity

Healthy Eating, Physical Activity, and Academic Performance

As of 2009, >95% of children and adolescents aged 5–17 years were enrolled in schools (*175*). Schools have direct contact with students for approximately 6 hours each day and for up to 13 critical years of their social, psychological, physical, and intellectual development (*176*). The health of students is strongly linked to their academic success, and the academic success of students is strongly linked with their health. Therefore, helping students stay healthy is a fundamental part of the mission of schools (*177–180*). School health programs and policies might be one of the most efficient means to prevent or reduce risk behaviors, prevent serious health problems among students, and help close the educational achievement gap (*181,182*). Schools offer an ideal setting for delivering health promotion strategies that provide opportunities for students to learn about and practice healthy behaviors. Schools, across all regional, demographic, and income categories, share the responsibility with families and communities to provide students with healthy environments that foster regular opportunities for healthy eating and physical activity. Healthy eating and physical activity also play a significant role in students' academic performance.

The importance of healthy eating, including eating breakfast, for the overall health and well-being of school-aged children cannot be understated. Most research on healthy eating and academic performance has focused on the negative effects of hunger and food insufficiency (*62*) and the importance of eating breakfast (*65,183,184*). Recent reviews of breakfast and cognition in students (*73,185,186*) report that eating a healthy breakfast might enhance cognitive function (especially memory), increase attendance rates, reduce absenteeism, and improve psychosocial function and mood. Certain improvements in academic performance such as improved math scores also were noted (*65,183*).

A growing body of research focuses on the association between school-based physical activity, including physical education, and academic performance among school-aged children and adolescents. A comprehensive CDC literature review that included 50 studies synthesized the scientific literature on the association between school-based physical activity, including physical education, and academic performance, including indicators of cognitive skills and attitudes, academic behaviors (e.g., concentration, attentiveness, and time on task), and academic achievement (e.g., grade point average and test scores). The review identified a total of 251 associations between school-based physical activity and academic performance. Of all the associations examined, 51% were positive, 48% were not significant, and 2% were negative. Therefore, the evidence suggests that 1) substantial evidence indicates that physical activity can help improve academic achievement, including grades and standardized test scores; 2) physical activity can affect cognitive skills and attitudes and academic behavior (including enhanced concentration, attention, and improved classroom behavior); and 3) increasing or maintaining time dedicated to physical education might help and does not appear to adversely affect academic performance (*187*).

Coordinated School Health Approach

Schools can promote the acquisition of lifelong healthy eating and physical activity behaviors through strategies that provide opportunities to practice and reinforce these behaviors. School efforts to promote healthy eating and physical activity should be part of a coordinated school health framework, which provides an integrated set of planned, sequential, and school-affiliated strategies, activities, and services designed to promote the optimal physical, emotional, social, and educational development of students. A coordinated school health framework involves families and is based on school and community needs, resources, and standards. The framework is coordinated by a multidisciplinary team such as a school health council and is accountable to the school and community for program quality and effectiveness (*182*).

School personnel, students, families, community organizations and agencies, and businesses can collaborate to successfully implement the coordinated school health approach and develop, implement, and evaluate healthy eating and physical activity efforts. Ideally, a coordinated school health framework integrates the efforts of eight components of the school environment that influence student health (i.e., comprehensive health education, physical education, and health services: mental health and social services, school nutrition services,

healthy and safe school environment, school employee wellness, and family and community involvement) (*188*). The following guidelines reflect the coordinated school health approach and include additional areas deemed to be important contributors to school health: policy development and implementation and professional development for program staff.

School Health Guidelines to Promote Healthy Eating and Physical Activity

This report includes nine general guidelines for school health programs to promote healthy eating and physical activity. Each guideline is followed by a series of strategies for implementing the general guidelines. Because each guideline is important to school health, there is no priority order. Guidelines presented first focus on the importance of a coordinated approach for nutrition and physical activity policies and practices within a health-promoting school environment. Then, guidelines pertaining to nutrition services and physical education are provided, followed by guidelines for health education, health, mental health and social services, family and community involvement, staff wellness, and professional development for staff.

Although the ultimate goal is to implement all guidelines recommended in this report, not every guideline and its corresponding strategies will be feasible for every school to implement. Because of resource limitations, some schools might need to implement the guidelines incrementally. Therefore, the recommendation is for schools to identify which guidelines are feasible to implement, based on the top health needs and priorities of the school and available resources. Families, school personnel, health-care providers, businesses, the media, religious organizations, community organizations that serve children and adolescents, and the students themselves also should be systematically involved in implementing the guidelines to optimize a coordinated approach to healthy eating and regular physical activity among school-aged children and adolescents.

The guidelines in this report are not clinical guidelines; compliance is neither mandatory nor tracked by CDC. However, CDC monitors the status of student health behaviors and school health policies and practices nationwide through three surveillance systems. These systems provide information about the degree to which students are participating in healthy behaviors and schools are developing and implementing the policies and practices recommended in the guidelines. The Youth Risk Behavior Surveillance System (YRBSS) monitors priority health-risk behaviors (e.g., unhealthy dietary behaviors and physical inactivity) and the prevalence of obesity and asthma among high school students. YRBSS includes a national, school-based survey conducted by CDC and state, territorial, tribal, and district surveys conducted by state, territorial, and local education and health agencies and tribal governments. YRBSS data are used to 1) measure progress toward achieving national health objectives for *Healthy People 2020* and other program and policy indicators, 2) assess trends in priority health-risk behaviors among adolescents and young adults, and 3) evaluate the effect of broad school and community interventions at the national, state, and local levels. In addition, state, territorial, and local agencies and nongovernmental organizations use YRBSS data to set and track progress toward meeting school health and health promotion program goals, support modification of school health curricula or other programs, support new legislation and policies that promote health, and seek funding and other support for new initiatives. The CDC School Health Policies and Practices Study (SHPPS) is a national survey conducted periodically to assess school health policies and practices at the state, district, school, and classroom levels. SHPPS data are used to 1) identify the characteristics of each school health program component (e.g., physical education and activity and nutrition services) at the state, district, school, and classroom (where applicable) levels across elementary, middle, and high schools; 2) identify persons responsible for coordinating and delivering each school health program component and their qualifications and educational background; 3) identify collaborations that occur among staff members from each school health program component and with staff members from outside agencies and organizations; and 4) describe changes in key policies and practices over time. The School Health Profiles (i.e., Profiles) is a system of surveys assessing school health policies and practices in states, large urban school districts, territories, and tribal governments. State, local, and territorial education and health officials use Profiles data to 1) describe school health policies and practices and compare them across jurisdictions, 2) identify professional development needs, 3) plan and monitor programs, 4) support health-related policies and legislation, 5) seek funding, and 6) garner support for future surveys. Results from the surveys are described throughout this report.

Guideline 1. Use a Coordinated Approach to Develop, Implement, and Evaluate Healthy Eating and Physical Activity Policies and Practices

Physical education, health education, and other teachers; school nutrition service staff members; school counselors; school nurses and other health, mental health, and social services staff members; community health-care providers; school administrators; student and parent groups; and community organizations should work together to maximize healthy eating and physical activity opportunities for students (Box 1). Coordination of all these persons and groups facilitates greater communication, minimizes duplication of policy and program initiatives, and increases the pooling of resources for healthy eating and physical activity policies and practices (*189–192*).

BOX 1. Strategies for guideline 1: Use a coordinated approach to develop, implement, and evaluate healthy eating and physical activity policies and practices

- Coordinate healthy eating and physical activity policies and practices through a school health council and school health coordinator.
- Assess healthy eating and physical activity policies and practices.
- Use a systematic approach to develop, implement, and monitor healthy eating and physical activity policies.
- Evaluate healthy eating and physical activity policies and practices.

Coordinate Healthy Eating and Physical Activity Policies and Practices Through a School Health Council and School Health Coordinator

Establish a school health council and designate a school health coordinator at the district level. Each district should have a school health council to help ensure that schools implement developmentally appropriate and evidence-based health policies and practices. Nationwide, in 2006, 73% of districts had one or more school health councils at the district level that offered guidance on the development of policies or coordinated activities on health topics (*193*). The school health council serves as a planning, advisory, and decision-making group for school health policies and programs. School health councils should include representatives from different segments of the school and community, including health and physical education teachers, nutrition service staff members, students, families, school administrators, school nurses and other health-care providers, social service professionals, and religious and civic leaders (*193–195*). The school health council provides input on decisions about how to promote health-enhancing behaviors, including healthy eating and physical activity among students. Some roles of school health councils include (*194*)

- needs assessment and resource mapping;
- program planning;
- advocacy;
- financial and resource planning;

- development of policies and practices, including those that address healthy eating and physical activity;
- assistance in reviewing and making recommendations about health-related curricula and instructional materials;
- communication of the importance of health and safety policies and activities to the superintendent, school board, schools, and community;
- coordination of school health programs and events within the school district and between schools and local community groups; and
- evaluation, accountability, and quality control of school health policies and programs.

Each district also should designate a school health coordinator who manages and coordinates health-related policies and practices across the district, including those related to healthy eating and physical activity. This person serves as an active member of the district-level school health council and communicates the district school health council's decisions and actions to school-level health coordinators and teams, staff, students, and parents (189,196–198). In 2006, 68% of districts had a person who oversaw or coordinated school health (e.g., a school health coordinator) (193). A district school health coordinator also should

- work closely with school-level health coordinators to ensure consistent implementation of health policies and practices across schools;
- coordinate professional development for school health staff members;
- secure funding and other resources to support school health and safety policies and activities;
- facilitate linkages between the district's health-related programs and services and health-related resources in the community; and
- coordinate evaluation of policies and practices.

Establish a school health team and designate a school health coordinator at the school level. Each school should establish a school health team, representative of school and community groups, to work with the greater school community to identify and address the health needs of students, school administrators, parents, and school staff. Nationwide, in 2006, 40% of schools had a school health council that offered guidance on the development of policies or coordinated activities on health topics (193). A school health team

- ensures that district-level policies and practices are implemented efficiently;
- communicates and coordinates with the district-level school health coordinator;
- assists with evaluating school health policies and practices;
- recommends new or revised health and safety policies and activities;

- assists in reviewing and making recommendations about health-related curricula and instructional materials;
- seeks funding or leverages resources to support school health and safety priorities; and
- communicates the importance of school health and safety policies and activities within the school, as well as to parents and the community.

Every school also should designate a school health coordinator to manage the school health policies, practices, activities, and resources, including those that address healthy eating and physical activity. In 2006, 61% of schools had someone at the school to oversee or coordinate school health (e.g., a school health coordinator) (193). School health coordinators might

- facilitate collaboration among school staff responsible for the health and safety of students;
- facilitate linkages between the school's health-related programs and services and health-related resources in the community (189,196,197);
- serve as a liaison between the school and those who oversee school health and safety programs at the district level and in other schools;
- communicate school health and safety priorities to the principal, staff, parents, community organizations, and students;
- help secure funding or other resources to support school building health and safety activities;
- manage school health funds;
- assist in the development of school health and safety policy materials and in the selection of educational materials;
- organize and conduct school health team meetings;
- facilitate the provision of professional development activities for school health staff; and
- assist with the assessment of student health needs and evaluation of school health policies and activities.

Assess Healthy Eating and Physical Activity Policies and Practices

An assessment of current school-based healthy eating and physical activity policies and practices is necessary to provide baseline information about strengths and weaknesses. An assessment can also identify how district-level policies are being implemented at the school level and in the development of community-specific strategies. An assessment enables the school health council, school health coordinator, parents, school administrators, and school board members to develop a data-based plan for improving student health. The CDC School Health Index: A Self-Assessment and Planning Guide (available at http://www.cdc.gov/healthyyouth/shi), a tool based on scientific evidence and best practices in school health, helps schools identify strengths and weaknesses of school policies and practices related to nutrition, physical activity, and other important health topics. Schools and school districts can refer to the School Health Index for a comprehensive list of policies and practices that promote healthy eating and physical activity in schools. The School Health Index guides schools through the development of an action plan to improve their school health policies and practices (*199,200*). Results from the School Health Index assessment and action plan can help schools determine where, what, and how to incorporate health promotion programs and policies into their overall school improvement plan. Inclusion in the school improvement plan helps ensure that health is a regular item on agendas of district school board meetings and school-based management committees.

Completing the School Health Index can lead to positive changes in the school health environment. For example, after completing the School Health Index, some schools have hired a physical education teacher for the first time, added healthier food choices to school meal programs, and incorporated structured fitness breaks into the school day (*201–203*). An assessment might also involve collection of data on current eating and physical activity behaviors of students, community-based nutrition and physical activity programs, and student, staff, and parent needs (*189*).

Use a Systematic Approach To Develop, Implement, and Monitor Healthy Eating and Physical Activity Policies

School health policies are official statements from education agencies and other governing bodies (e.g., state legislatures) at the state, district, or school level. They identify what should be done, why it should be done, and who is responsible for doing it. School health policies can (*204*)

- provide evidence of leadership, commitment, and support for school health, including healthy eating and physical activity, from school boards, school administrators, and other decision makers;
- drive positive changes in healthy eating and physical activity programs;
- sustain and expand healthy eating and physical activity programs or activities;
- establish accountability by identifying who is responsible for healthy eating and physical activity programs and policies; and
- establish performance measures.

School health policies should comply with federal, state, and local laws and mandates. School health councils, teams, and coordinators can lead the development, implementation, and monitoring of policies (*194,196*).

The Child Nutrition and WIC Reauthorization Act of 2004 required that each school district participating in the federally supported meal program establish a local school wellness policy for the first time by school year 2006 (*205*). By 2007–2008, most school districts had a local wellness policy; however, the quality of policies varied across school districts. In addition, many of the policies lacked plans for implementing and monitoring the status of the wellness policy (*206*).

The Healthy, Hunger-Free Kids Act of 2010 (*207*) updated requirements for local school wellness policy to include, at a minimum,

- goals for nutrition promotion and education, physical activity, and other school-based activities that promote student wellness;
- nutrition guidelines for all foods available on each school campus under the jurisdiction of the local educational agency during the school day that are consistent with requirements in the act and that promote student health and reduce childhood obesity;
- a requirement that the local education agency permit parents, students, representatives of the school food authority, teachers of physical education, school health professionals, the school board, school administrators, and the general public to participate in the development, implementation, and periodic review and update of the local school wellness policy;
- a requirement that the local education agency inform and update the public on local school wellness policy content and implementation;
- a requirement that the local education agency periodically measure and make available to the public an assessment on the implementation of the local school wellness policy, including the level of school implementation, how the local school wellness policy compares with model policy, and a description of progress made toward goals; and
- a requirement that the local education agency designate one or more local education agency officials or school officials to ensure that each school complies with the local school wellness policy.

The act also requires that the U.S. Department of Agriculture (USDA), in conjunction with the CDC director, "prepare a report on the implementation, strength, and effectiveness of the local school wellness policies" (*207*).

States, districts, and schools should use a systematic approach when developing, implementing, and monitoring healthy eating and physical activity policies. They can use the following strategies throughout the policy process.

Identify and involve key stakeholders from the beginning of the policy process. One person, such as the school health coordinator (at the district or school level, depending on the level at which the policy is to be implemented), should assume or be designated with overall responsibility for coordinating and implementing healthy eating and physical activity policies. This person also can help identify and involve key stakeholders, including the school health council or team. Key stakeholders in district- and school-level policy processes include students, families, school nutrition service staff, physical education teachers, health education teachers, school nurses, school principals and other administrators, staff from local health departments, health-care providers, and staff from local community organizations and businesses. This group of stakeholders will contribute to the development, implementation, and monitoring of healthy eating and physical activity policies.

Draft the policy language. Policy language should be specific, simple, clear, and accurate; avoid education, health, and legal jargon; and be easy for readers with diverse backgrounds to understand and apply. Policy language should be consistent with state, district, and school visions for student learning and health and other policies in the same jurisdiction. A written policy should describe (*204*)

- who establishes the policy and the underlying legal authority;
- the rationale for the policy, including emphasis on the effects of health on academic achievement;
- the priority population (e.g., students and school staff members) to which the policy applies;
- definitions of key terms;
- a list and descriptions of the major activities to be conducted;
- who will be responsible for implementing the policy;
- who will enforce the policy and how they will do so;
- positive incentives for compliance and consequences for noncompliance;
- an evaluation plan, including how the effect of the policy will be measured and how the evaluation information will be used; and
- a timeline indicating when the policy will be adopted, take effect, and expire.

Resources to guide policy development include the National Association of State Boards of Education's (NASBE's) *Fit, Healthy, and Ready to Learn* (*204*), USDA's local wellness policy website (*208*), and the Action for Healthy Kids policy development tool (*209*). NASBE's state school health policy database includes a comprehensive set of laws and policies from 50 states on approximately 40 school health topics (available at http://www.nasbe.org/healthy_schools/hs).

Adopt, implement, and monitor healthy eating and physical activity policies. After the draft policy is completed, the process of adopting the policy begins (*204,210*). To ensure greater support for policy adoption, school health council members or other policy makers should be given time to share the draft policy with their partners and gather reactions. Public hearings or other meetings that gather wider input from the school and community might be beneficial or required. Such hearings allow every interested person or organization to provide input on the policy.

Policy adoption typically requires that the drafted policy be presented to the policy-making body (e.g., the school board or school administrators). The presentation should include background information about why the policy is needed (e.g., data about the eating and physical activity habits of students) and concise information about the policy. Policies likely will require final approval by the school board, the district superintendent, or both.

Implementation of policies should be a cooperative effort that includes the school health coordinator, school health council, and school staff members. All school staff members and teachers, in particular, need sufficient time to implement the policy and make agreed-on changes in the school environment to support the policy (*211*). Those responsible for implementation should be prepared to address challenges, such as perceptions that the policy is low priority, limited resources for full implementation, changes in school administrators and school staff members, and concerns such as lost revenue from certain food and beverage sales and resolving scheduling conflicts for use of physical activity facilities because of increasing numbers of physical activity programs (*210*). Parental and community concerns might be mitigated by making incremental changes and ensuring that the media receive positive stories about the response to the policy. Monitoring policy implementation allows school staff members to determine whether the policy yielded the expected results and which changes could be made to improve the results.

Establishing policy is an important component of many of the nine guidelines. Following is a list of key healthy eating and physical activity policies that are described in the remaining guidelines:

- Provide nutritious and appealing school meals that comply with the U.S. *Dietary Guidelines for Americans*.
- Ensure that foods and beverages sold or served outside of school meal programs follow the *Dietary Guidelines for Americans* and are consistent with the most recent scientific guidelines for nutrition standards.
- Require daily planned and sequential physical education from grades K–12.
- Require daily recess for elementary schools.
- Require planned and sequential health education from prekindergarten through grade 12.

- Require physical education specialists, health education specialists, and certified food service staff members to be hired for grades K–12.
- Provide school staff members with comprehensive professional development to deliver quality health education, physical education, food services, and health services.

Evaluate Healthy Eating and Physical Activity Policies and Practices

Evaluation can be used to assess and improve policies and practices that promote increased physical activity and healthier eating among students and faculty members. All groups involved in and affected by school efforts to promote lifelong physical activity and healthy eating should have the opportunity to contribute to evaluation. Education agencies and schools should designate a person to take the lead on evaluation activities. Schools may choose to enlist local universities, the health department, or the education department to assist with the evaluation of school policies and practices.

Evaluation can serve various purposes, including 1) improving the content, support for, and implementation of physical activity and healthy eating policies and practices; 2) documenting changes in the school environment, physical education and health education curricula, physical activity and healthy eating services for students and school staff members, physical activity and dietary habits, and health outcomes such as blood pressure and blood glucose levels; 3) identifying strengths and weakness of policies and practices and making a plan for improvement; and 4) responding to new and changing needs of students and school staff members. Although evaluations should not be used to audit or rank schools or penalize school staff members (*199,200*), evaluations can be used to motivate schools to make changes and monitor school-level implementation of school district, state, and federal policies.

Two fundamental types of evaluation are process and outcome. In process evaluation, educators collect and analyze data to determine who, what, when, where, and how much of program activities have been conducted. Process evaluation is the foundation of evaluation because it specifies the activities involved in policies, programs, and practices, and whether they were implemented as intended. In addition, process evaluation allows education agency staff members to assess how well a policy, program, or practice has been implemented and what strengths and improvements are necessary.

Outcome evaluation explores whether intended outcomes or specific changes occur as a direct result of policies, programs, or practices. Outcomes might include changes at the school level (e.g., changes in school environment, norms, or curricula) and at the individual level (e.g., student knowledge, attitudes, skills, and behaviors). Outcome evaluation can require a great deal of time, money, and expertise, and individual schools are unlikely to be able to conduct outcome evaluations on their own. A full-fledged outcome evaluation might be beyond the reach of most schools and is more likely the purview of state and local education agencies. However, some outcome-related questions can be answered using simple methods available to most schools. Outcome evaluation can focus on short- or long-term outcomes of policies, programs, or practices, including changes in practices at the school level or changes in student knowledge, attitudes, skills, behaviors, or health outcomes.

Conduct process evaluation of nutrition and physical activity policies and practices. Schools should conduct a process evaluation of their healthy eating and physical activity policies and practices. Process evaluation topics for schools might include the following:

- Did schools establish a school health council and conduct an assessment of their existing healthy eating and physical activity policies and practices?
- Did schools communicate about the development, implementation, and monitoring of healthy eating and physical activity policies to school administrators, school staff members, and others affected by the policies?
- Did schools develop a communications and marketing plan to promote participation in school breakfast, lunch, and other feeding programs that provide foods consistent with the *Dietary Guidelines for Americans*?
- Did schools provide training to physical education teachers on instructional strategies that would keep all students active for most of physical education class time?

Conduct outcome evaluation of healthy eating and physical activity policies, programs, and practices. In addition to the process evaluation topics, schools might evaluate changes that occurred after a policy, program, or practice was implemented. Outcome evaluation topics include the following:

- Did all foods and beverages sold in school stores, vending machines, and a la carte lines adhere to strong nutrition standards for all foods in schools?
- Did students' consumption of fruits and vegetables increase after their school increased the availability of fruits and vegetables?
- Did all students in all grades participate in daily recess throughout the school year?
- Did students' levels of physical activity increase after they participated in physical education?

CDC's *Framework for Program Evaluation in Public Health* summarizes and organizes essential elements of program evaluation (*212*). The *Physical Activity Evaluation Handbook* illustrates the six steps of program evaluation in the framework with physical activity program examples (*213*). *Understanding*

Evaluation: The Way to Better Prevention Programs describes evaluation activities that school districts and community agencies can use to assess various programs (*214*). State and local education agencies and schools can consult with evaluators at universities, school districts, or state departments of education and health to identify methods and materials for evaluating their efforts.

Guideline 2. Establish School Environments that Support Healthy Eating and Physical Activity

The physical surroundings and psychosocial climate of a school should encourage all students to make healthy eating choices and be physically active. The physical environment includes the entire school building and the area surrounding it; facilities for physical activity, physical education, and food preparation and consumption; availability of food and physical activity options; and conditions such as temperature, air quality, noise, lighting, and safety (*215*). The psychosocial environment includes the social norms established by policies and practices that influence the physical activity and eating behaviors of students and staff members (*216*). Developing and maintaining a supportive school environment can improve the sustainability of healthy eating and physical activity policies and practices that support healthy lifestyles (*147,217,218*) (Box 2).

Provide Access to Healthy Foods and Physical Activity Opportunities and to Safe Spaces, Facilities, and Equipment for Healthy Eating and Physical Activity

Provide adequate and safe spaces and facilities for healthy eating. Students should have access to a well-maintained cafeteria that is clean, is pleasant, has appropriate seating arrangements, and does not exceed 100% capacity (*215,219–221*). School nutrition services should serve healthy food in an environment that allows students to pay attention to what they are eating and enjoy social aspects of dining (*215,220–223*). Students can enjoy meal time more when they feel relaxed and are able to socialize without feeling rushed. Actions to support safe and healthy eating include

- ensuring sufficient time to receive and consume a meal, with at least 10 minutes for eating breakfast and 20 minutes for eating lunch after being seated (*215,224*);
- providing recess before lunch, which can reduce plate waste, increase student consumption of food (*225*), decrease student wait time in line, and reduce student discipline referrals (*226*);

BOX 2. Strategies for guideline 2: Establish school environments that support healthy eating and physical activity

- Provide access to healthy foods and physical activity opportunities and to safe spaces, facilities, and equipment for healthy eating and physical activity.
- Establish a climate that encourages and does not stigmatize healthy eating and physical activity.
- Create a school environment that encourages a healthy body image, shape, and size among all students and staff members, is accepting of diverse abilities, and does not tolerate weight-based teasing.

- providing opportunities for students to wash or sanitize their hands in a convenient place before eating;
- providing tables and chairs of appropriate size, with space to accommodate all students with special needs (e.g., students who use wheel chairs and students with food allergies);
- maintaining an appropriate ambient noise level using acceptable and positive enforcement practices (e.g., no whistles and no orders to eat in silence [silent lunch]); and
- implementing rules for safe behavior.

Other food environment activities, such as school gardens, school salad bars, and farm-to-school programs, can enrich the eating and educational experience by providing quality produce and opportunities for hands-on multidisciplinary learning (*227–231*). In 2002, the National School Lunch Act (*232*) was amended with a provision encouraging institutions participating in the school lunch and breakfast programs "to purchase unprocessed agricultural products, both locally grown and locally raised, to the maximum extent practicable and appropriate" (*233*). In addition to integrating local agriculture products, such as fruits, vegetables, and eggs, into the school cafeteria, farm-to-school activities include hands-on education through school garden programs and field trips to local farms, classroom nutrition education, and alternative fundraising using local produce (*234*). School garden programs have the potential to strengthen the healthy development of students through improved knowledge about fruits and vegetables (*228,231,235*), increased preference for fruits and vegetables (*228,231,235*), and increased consumption of fruits and vegetables (*230,231,235,236*).

Schools also should ensure that students have access to safe, free, and well-maintained drinking water fountains or dispensers during school meals, as required by the Healthy, Hunger-Free Kids Act (*237*), as well as throughout the school day (*238*). This provides a healthy alternative to sugar-sweetened beverages and can help increase students' overall water consumption (*239,240*). The National Policy and Legal Analysis Network (NPLAN) to Prevent Childhood Obesity has resources for developing policies and best practices to increase access to free drinking water in schools (available at http://www.nplanonline.org/childhood-obesity/products/water-access).

Ensure that spaces and facilities for physical activity meet or exceed recommended safety standards. The following should be in place to support safe and enjoyable student physical activity: 1) safe and age-appropriate playgrounds and equipment for physical education, physical activity, and recess during the school day (*187,241–244*); 2) safe routes to school, particularly for students living ≤1 mile from school (*110*); and 3) access to extracurricular programs such as intramurals and interscholastic sports that are age appropriate, are safe, provide proper equipment when needed, and are available for all students (*241,242,245,246*).

All spaces and facilities for physical activity, including playing fields, playgrounds, gymnasiums, swimming pools, multipurpose rooms, cafeterias, and fitness centers, should be regularly inspected and maintained, hazardous conditions should be corrected immediately, and a comprehensive safety assessment should be done at least annually (*247,248*). Regular inspection and maintenance of indoor and outdoor play surfaces should ensure that environmental safety devices are provided and maintained, including (*244,248*)

- padded goal posts (*249*) and gym walls;
- breakaway bases for baseball and softball (*250,251*);
- slip-resistant surfaces near swimming pools;
- sidewalks that are clear of debris and other hazards;
- securely anchored portable soccer goals that are stored in a locked facility when not in use;
- shade structures that are used for sun safety;
- bleachers that minimize the risk for falls; and
- pools and spas designed, constructed, and retrofitted to eliminate entrapment hazards (including evisceration or disembowelment, body entrapment, and hair entrapment or entanglement).

Develop, teach, implement, and enforce safety rules. Safe physical activity requires proper conditioning and use of appropriate equipment where needed. Dangerous behaviors (e.g., spearing in football, high-sticking in hockey, throwing a bat in baseball, and use of alcohol and other drugs by athletes) can be prohibited by establishing and enforcing rules (*252,253*). Explicit safety rules should be taught to and followed by students in physical education, extracurricular physical activity programs, and community sports and recreation programs (*244,246,254*). Adult supervisors should consistently reinforce safety rules, which should be posted in

key locations. One person, such as the school health coordinator or lead physical education teacher, should be responsible for ensuring that safety measures are in place and updated as needed (*198,255*); however, minimizing physical activity–related injuries and illnesses among children and adolescents is the joint responsibility of teachers, administrators, coaches, athletic trainers, school nurses, other school and community personnel, parents, and students (*254,256*).

Maintain high levels of supervision during structured and unstructured physical activity programs. Trained staff members or volunteers, including coaches, teachers, parents, paraprofessionals, and community members, should supervise all physical activity programs. Staff members should be aware of the potential for physical activity–related injuries and illnesses among students so that the risks for and consequences of these injuries and illnesses can be minimized. To prevent injuries during structured physical activity schools can

- require physical assessment before participation (*257*);
- provide developmentally appropriate activities (*246*);
- ensure proper conditioning and avoid excesses in training (*258–260*);
- provide student instruction regarding the biomechanics of specific motor skills (*260*);
- appropriately match participants according to size and ability;
- adapt rules to the skill level of students and the protective equipment available (*259*);
- modify rules to eliminate unsafe practices;
- ensure that injuries, including concussions, are healed before allowing further participation; and
- establish criteria, including clearance by a health-care provider, for reentering play after an injury to ensure that injuries are fully healed.

Children and adolescents also could be provided with, and required to use, protective clothing and equipment appropriate for the type of physical activity and the environment (*259*). Protective clothing and equipment includes footwear appropriate for the specific activity; helmets for bicycling; helmets, face masks, mouth guards, and protective pads for football and ice hockey; shin guards for soccer; knee pads for in-line skating; and reflective clothing for walking and running. As a general recommendation, all protective equipment should 1) be in good condition; 2) be inspected and maintained frequently; 3) be replaced if worn, damaged, or outdated; 4) provide a good fit for the athlete; and 5) be appropriate for the sport and position. In addition, children and adolescents need to be trained to use equipment correctly; this is particularly true of helmets (*261*).

To prevent injuries during unstructured play time, schools should consider implementing training sessions for staff members focusing on observation techniques, behavior management, appropriate supervision, and emergency response procedures (*244*). Additional information that schools might want to integrate into training sessions can be found in the *Consumer Product Safety Commission Handbook for Public Playground Safety* (*243*). In general, playground supervisors should 1) repetitively teach children playground rules; 2) prevent, recognize, and stop children's dangerous and risky behavior; 3) help children to identify, acknowledge, and prevent their risky behavior; and 4) model appropriate safety behavior (*243,262*). When possible, schools can support those supervising unstructured physical activity by following the National Program for Playground Safety (NPPS) recommendations that the playground supervision ratio of teachers to students be equal to the indoor classroom ratio (*263*).

Increase community access to school physical activity facilities. Schools should provide community access to physical activity facilities, such as gymnasiums, tracks, baseball and softball fields, basketball courts, outdoor play areas, and indoor fitness centers during the school day and out-of-school time (*242,264,265*). In 2006, adults used school physical activity or athletic facilities during out-of-school–time hours for community-sponsored sports teams in 47% of all schools, for open gym in 31% of schools, and for physical activity classes or lessons in 23% of schools (*144*).

Establishing a formal policy or agreement, such as a joint use agreement, between schools and community organizations can help increase student, family, and community access to physical activity facilities and programs. A joint use agreement is a policy that allows two or more entities (e.g., schools, community organizations) to share use of their facilities. Joint use agreements provide details about the facilities to be shared, as well as scheduling, management, maintenance, and costs of the shared facilities. Roles, responsibilities, and liability terms also are typically outlined within joint use agreements (*266*). Access to these facilities can help to increase visibility of schools, provide community members a safe place for physical activity, and might increase partnerships with community-based physical activity programs (*266,267*). The National Policy and Legal Analysis Network to Prevent Childhood Obesity (available at http://www.nplanonline.org/nplan/joint-use) and the Prevention Institute (available at http://www.jointuse.org) offer free resources to assess school facilities for community use and establish joint use agreements.

Frequently, schools have the facilities but lack the personnel to deliver extracurricular physical activity programs. Community resources can expand existing school programs by providing program staff members as well as intramural and club activities on school grounds. For example, community agencies and organizations can use school facilities

for after-school physical fitness programs for students, weight management programs for overweight or obese students, and sports and recreation programs for students with disabilities or chronic health conditions.

Establish a Climate that Encourages and Does Not Stigmatize Healthy Eating and Physical Activity

Adopt marketing techniques to promote healthy dietary choices. Marketing techniques can be used to promote healthy foods and beverages among students. The following techniques have been used in schools to increase the likelihood of students choosing healthier foods and beverages:

- placing nutritious products so that they are easy for students to choose, such as featuring fruits and vegetables, low-fat and fat-free milk and other dairy products, and whole grains in prominent places in cafeteria lines (*268*)
- promoting healthy eating through environmental strategies such as prompts, parental outreach, and point-of-purchase promotions (*269,270*) because point-of-purchase signage and parental newsletters highlighting parents' healthy eating behaviors influence children's food selections (*269,271*)
- applying pricing strategies, such as lowering the price of nutritious items and, if offered, raising the price of less nutritious items, because this practice encourages students to purchase more healthy items (*269,272–274*)

Use student rewards that support health. Student achievement or positive classroom behavior should only be rewarded with nonfood items or activities. In 2006, only 17% of all schools prohibited faculty and staff members from using food or food coupons as a reward for good behavior or good academic performance (*105*). The use of food as rewards, especially foods with little nutritional value, might increase the risk that children associate such foods with emotions, such as feelings of accomplishment (*268,275*). Providing food based on performance or behavior connects the experience of eating food to the student's perceptions and mood. Rewarding students with food during class also reinforces eating outside of meal or snack times. This practice can encourage students to eat treats even when they are not hungry and instill lifetime habits of rewarding or comforting themselves with unhealthy eating, resulting in overconsumption of foods high in added sugar and fat (*276–278*). Although few studies have examined the effect of using food rewards on students' long-term eating habits, the IOM Nutrition Standards for Foods in Schools report determined that such use of foods in schools is inappropriate (*238*) because this practice establishes an emotional connection between foods and accomplishments.

When an extrinsic reward system is used, rewards should be nonfood items or activities (e.g., stickers, books, or extra time for recess) to recognize students for their achievements or good behavior. The Center for Science in the Public Interest lists examples of constructive student rewards (available at http://cspinet.org/new/pdf/constructive_classroom_rewards.pdf).

Do not use physical activity as punishment. Teachers, coaches, and other school and community personnel should not use physical activity as punishment or withhold opportunities for physical activity as a form of punishment. Nationwide in 2006, in 32% of schools, school staff members were allowed to use physical activity (e.g., running laps or doing push-ups) to punish students for bad behavior in physical education. In 23% of schools, staff members were allowed to exclude students from all or part of physical education as punishment for bad behavior in another class (*144*). Using physical activity as a punishment (e.g., forcing students to perform push-ups or sit-ups for bad behavior in physical education) might create negative associations with physical activity in the minds of students (*279*). Exclusion from physical education or recess for bad behavior in a classroom deprives students of physical activity experiences that benefit health and can contribute toward improved behavior in the classroom (*280,281*). Disciplining students for unacceptable behavior or academic performance by not allowing them to participate in recess or physical education prevents students from 1) accumulating valuable free-time physical activity and 2) learning essential physical activity knowledge and skills.

Create a School Environment that Encourages a Healthy Body Image, Shape, and Size Among All Students and Staff Members, Is Accepting of Diverse Abilities, and Does Not Tolerate Weight-Based Teasing

The psychological environment at a school should support all students in making healthy eating choices and being physically active, regardless of race/ethnicity, income, sex, and physical ability (*215*). Schools can take numerous steps to help shape a health-promoting psychological environment. For example, they can adopt and enforce a universal bullying prevention program that addresses weight discrimination and teasing (*215,282,283*), ensure that students of all sizes are encouraged to participate in a wide variety of physical activities (*279*), display posters or other visual materials that feature a diverse combination of students being active and eating healthy, and avoid practices that single out students on the basis of body size or shape (*283*). Schools should avoid elimination games such as dodge ball, bombardment, and elimination tag that limit opportunities for all students to be active (*284*). School health, mental health, and social services staff members can play a key role in helping to communicate and promote these practices.

The school nutrition policy should ensure a safe environment for students with chronic health conditions. The policy should cover all venues where foods and beverages are available, during the regular and extended school day, and all families and staff members should be informed of the policy (*215*). Nutrition service staff members should be provided with information and support to assist students who are on nutrition programs or diets prescribed by their health-care provider. USDA provides guidance on accommodating children with special dietary needs, supported by the USDA nondiscrimination regulation (*285*), allowing for substitutions or modifications in the National School Meals Program for children whose disabilities restrict their diet as certified by a licensed physician (*286*). The school nutrition service staff members also should consider making food substitutions for students with food allergies, for students with food intolerances, or on a case-by-case basis for students who are medically certified as having a special medical dietary need (*286*).

The school environment should support students with disabilities and chronic health conditions in being physically active and making healthy eating choices. A chronic health condition is defined as any illness, disease, disorder, or disability of long duration or frequent recurrence, including asthma, diabetes, serious allergies, epilepsy, and obesity (*287*). Schools should establish policies that allow full participation by all students in physical activity, including extracurricular activities, and ensure access to preventive and quick-relief medications as indicated by a student's Individualized Health Care Plan, 504 plan, Individualized Education Plan (IEP), or all of these as appropriate (*204,288–297*). Coordination between health services staff members, special education, nutrition services staff members, and health and physical education staff members can help ensure that these policies are established.

Guideline 3. Provide a Quality School Meal Program and Ensure that Students Have Only Appealing, Healthy Food and Beverage Choices Offered Outside of the School Meal Program

Schools are in a unique position to promote healthy dietary behaviors and help ensure appropriate food and nutrient intake among their students. Many schools provide students with access to foods and beverages in various venues across the school campus, including meals served in the cafeteria as part of the federally reimbursable school meal program and competitive foods (i.e., foods and beverages that are sold, served, or given to students but are not part of the school meal program). Schools should model and reinforce healthy dietary behaviors by ensuring that only nutritious and appealing foods and beverages are provided in all venues accessible to students (Box 3).

Promote Access to and Participation in School Meals

Schools should provide students with access to breakfast, lunch, and other important programs (e.g., after-school snack programs and summer feeding programs) and promote participation in these programs by all students (*298,299*). A school meal program offers students the opportunity to apply knowledge and skills learned through nutrition education, can affect students' food choices by providing nutrient information of the foods available, and can encourage students to make healthy choices (*98,300,301*).

The USDA's Food and Nutrition Service administers the federally sponsored school meal programs including the National School Lunch Program and the School Breakfast Program. Although schools are not required to participate in these programs, 94% of schools, both public and private, participate in the National School Lunch Program (*68*). Among public schools offering the National School Lunch Program, approximately 81% also offer the School Breakfast Program (*302*). School districts and independent schools that choose to take part in the federal school meal programs receive cash reimbursements and entitlement funds for USDA Foods (commodities), provided that the meals they serve meet federal requirements and that they offer free or reduced price lunches to eligible students.

The School Breakfast Program and National School Lunch Program play major roles in the diets of children and adolescents in the United States. Approximately 30 million students participate in the National School Lunch Program every school day, with approximately 63% of school lunches served free or at a reduced price for students from low-income families (*303*). An average of 10 million children participate in the School Breakfast Program each school day, and 82% of these breakfasts are provided free or at a reduced price to students from low-income families (*304*). On a typical school day during the 2004–2005 school year, among students who participated in both the School Breakfast Program and the National School Lunch Program, an average of 47% of their calories came from meals and snacks consumed at school (*305*). Students who participate in school meal programs have been found to consume more milk, fruits, and vegetables and have better nutrient intake than those who do not participate (*306,307*). However, participants in the School Breakfast Program and National School Lunch Program also have higher sodium intake from school meals than those who do not participate (*308*). In addition, regular participation in the School Breakfast Program is associated with lower BMI among students (*309*).

Student participation in school meal programs, particularly breakfast, has been shown to be associated in the short term with improved student functioning on a broad range of psychosocial and academic measures (*65,310–312*). Studies of students who participated more often in school breakfast programs showed increases in test scores and significant decreases in the rates of school absence and tardiness compared with students whose participation remained the same or decreased (*65,313*).

Encourage participation in school meal programs among all students. Participation rates in school meal programs vary by sex, income, age, and race/ethnicity. In the 2004–2005 school year, boys participated in the National School Lunch Program at a higher rate than girls, elementary school students participated at a higher rate than middle and high school students, students who were eligible for free and reduced-price meals participated at a higher rate than students who were not income eligible, rural students participated at a higher rate than urban students, and students whose parents did not attend college participated at a higher rate than those parents who did. In the 2004–2005 school year, boys participated in the School Breakfast Program at a higher rate than girls, non-Hispanic black students participated at a higher rate than Hispanic students and non-Hispanic white students, elementary school students participated at a higher rate than middle and high school students, students who were eligible for free and reduced-price meals participated at a higher rate than students who were not income eligible, students who spoke Spanish in the home participated at a higher rate than students who spoke English, and rural students participated at a higher rate than urban students (*314*). Participation decreased as grade level increased, decreasing from 73% among elementary students to 60% among middle school students and 44% among high school (*314*).

All students are eligible to participate in the school meal program; however, schools receive a smaller reimbursement for students who exceed income limits than for students from low-income families. Increased effort is needed to ensure that participation in a school meal program that complies with the *Dietary Guidelines for Americans* is promoted and supported.

To encourage increased participation in school meal programs by all students, schools can use the following strategies:

- Offer breakfast to all students at no cost to increase overall participation in the school breakfast program (*315*).
- Offer breakfast through alternative service methods (e.g., breakfast carts, breakfast in the classroom, breakfast after first period, and "grab and go").
- Use Provision 2 and Provision 3 (*316*) of the National School Lunch Act to reduce paperwork and applications and to simplify meal counting and claiming procedures. Schools using Provision 2 and Provision 3 establish claiming percentages for reimbursement and serve meals free to all participating students for 4 years.
- Use direct certification to automatically qualify students who participate in Temporary Assistance to Needy Families, the Supplemental Nutrition Assistance Program (formerly the Food Stamp Program), and the Food Distribution Program on Indian Reservations for free meals without requiring additional applications.
- Eliminate the reduced-price category for breakfast. This option, as well as direct certification, Provision 2 and Provision 3, and alternate service methods are described in USDA Food and Nutrition Service School Breakfast Toolkit (available at http://www.fns.usda.gov/cnd/breakfast/expansion).
- Eliminate any social stigma attached to, and prevent the overt identification of, students who are eligible for free and reduced-price school meals (*317*).
- Ensure that meals meet students' cultural preferences; for example, encourage students and parents to participate in planning meals and incorporating cultural and regional preferences.
- Obtain input from students about menu choices through taste-testing and the school health council.
- Serve meals at an appropriate time, such as 11:00 a.m.– 1:00 p.m., in a supportive, comfortable, and attractive environment with a minimal wait time (*222*).
- Have school nutrition staff members and teachers collaborate to design and implement nutrition education programs that promote healthy eating messages to the entire school community (*299*).

Provide Nutritious and Appealing School Meals that Comply with the *Dietary Guidelines for Americans*

The school meal program should provide various healthy, appetizing, and culturally appropriate choices to help students meet their nutritional needs. Meals served in the National School Lunch Program and School Breakfast Program must meet federally defined nutrition standards based on the *Dietary Guidelines for Americans* for schools to be eligible for federal subsidies. On average per week, current school lunches must have no more than 30% of calories from fat, with <10% from saturated fat, and must provide one third of the Recommended Dietary Allowances of protein, vitamin A, vitamin C, iron, calcium, and calories. Decisions about the specific foods to offer and how to prepare them are made by local school food authorities. The Healthy, Hunger-Free Kids Act of 2010 requires USDA to update the meal patterns and nutrition standards for the National School Lunch Program and School Breakfast Program based on recommendations made by the Food and Nutrition Board of the National Research Council of the National Academies of Sciences (*318*). The 2009 IOM report *School Meals: Building Blocks for Healthy Children* (*319*) recommendations reflect current dietary guidance including increasing the requirements for fruits, vegetables and whole grains, requiring only fat-free and low-fat milk, and decreasing the amount of sodium and trans fat in school meals. Schools that provide meals that meet these recommendations will receive an additional $0.06 (6 cents) for each qualifying meal served (*318*).

Schools also should take necessary action to prevent or minimize the risk for foodborne illness among participants in the National School Lunch Program and School Breakfast Program. School food authorities are required to develop and implement a food safety program based on a hazard analysis critical control point system (*320*). This law allows school food authorities to identify potential food hazards, identify critical points where hazards can be eliminated or minimized through control measures, and establish monitoring procedures and corrective action. The National Food Service Management Institute and USDA's Food and Nutrition Service offer various trainings and resources to assist school food authorities in implementing food safety programs.

Ensure that meals meet federally defined nutrition standards. Schools have made considerable progress in meeting federal nutrition requirements for school meals. A national study conducted during the 2004–2005 school year found that approximately 85% of public schools offering the National School Lunch Program served meals that met the standards for protein, vitamins, and minerals; 88% offered a vegetable (not including French fries) every day; 50% offered fresh fruit every day; and 62% offered canned fruit every day (*306,321*). However, although three fourths of schools met the fat standards in school breakfasts, less than one third of schools met the standards for calories from fat or saturated fat in the average lunch (*321*). For both breakfast and lunch, average levels of sodium were higher and fiber was lower than the *Dietary Guidelines for Americans* recommendations (*321*).

Schools can choose to take USDA's Healthier U.S. School Challenge to create healthier food and beverage choices. Schools that engage in the Healthier U.S. School Challenge commit to meeting specified criteria including stricter nutrition standards such as increasing the number of servings of whole-grain foods, dark green and orange vegetables, and dry beans and peas.

The USDA *A Menu Planner for Healthy School Meals* provides information on how to plan, prepare, serve, and market healthy school meals (*322*). School nutrition services staff members may modify menus to include healthier foods, such as serving more fruits, vegetables, and whole grains, and offering a greater variety of low-fat foods, including fat-free and low-fat milk. Other ideas include serving foods such as salsas for fresh flavor and less fat; making reductions and substitutions, such as reducing salt and using low-fat mayonnaise and salad dressings; and preparing foods in different ways, such as baking rather than frying French fries or serving baked potatoes instead (*322,323*).

Ensure that schools have kitchen facilities and equipment needed to cook quality, appealing meals. Support should be provided to schools to upgrade kitchen facilities with state-of-the-art equipment, which can help ensure that school meals are appealing to children and that they are prepared using the most healthy cooking techniques and food products available. Serving baked instead of fried foods can make a substantial difference in the amount of calories, fat, and saturated fat that children consume. For example, baked French fries have 55% less total fat and 34% less saturated fat than deep-fried French fries (*324*). Ovens, instead of deep-fat fryers, are needed to bake fries, but not all schools have such equipment and need financial support to purchase these types of items (*190,325,326*).

Outdated kitchen equipment, limited and inadequate kitchen facilities, and food budgets are substantial barriers for school nutrition staff members to provide healthy and appealing school meals (*323,327–330*). Recent trends associated with the need to update kitchen equipment in school nutrition programs include an increased emphasis on health and wellness, food security and emergency preparedness, smaller and more mobile equipment (e.g., for salad bars), blended technologies (e.g., combination oven-steamers), and machines that vend complete reimbursable school meals (*331*). The National Food Service Management Institute (available at http://www.nfsmi.org) offers training and resources on effective equipment purchasing guidance and financial management practices of operating a school nutrition program.

Use healthy food preparation methods and purchasing techniques. Healthy food preparation methods play an important role in providing nutritious and appealing meals

and include practices such as substitution techniques (i.e., substituting one type of ingredient for another), reduction techniques (i.e., reducing the amount of an ingredient), fat-reduction techniques when preparing meat and poultry, and vegetable preparation techniques. When making substitutions or reductions in ingredients, schools should standardize the recipe to account for the changes in yield and meal pattern requirements. Standardized recipes help to ensure that the products are prepared consistently, provide a defined yield, and list the meal pattern contribution. Schools should seek out and taste test standardized recipes that are low in fat, oil, salt, and sugar to ensure that they are acceptable to students. Schools may consider USDA Foods (commodities), which have been modified to reduce sodium and fat, including saturated fat, as substitutions for less healthy ingredients.

Substitution techniques include the following (*5,105,332*):
- Use cooked dry beans, canned beans, soybeans, or other meat extenders instead of meat.
- Use ground turkey or lean ground beef instead of regular ground beef.
- Use low-fat or fat-free yogurt, mayonnaise, or sour cream instead of regular mayonnaise, sour cream, or creamy salad dressings.
- Use frozen vegetables or low-sodium canned vegetables instead of regular canned vegetables.
- Use frozen fruits or canned fruits packed in juice instead of canned fruits packed in syrup.
- Use nonstick spray or pan liners instead of grease or oil.
- Use seasonings other than salt.
- Use part-skim or low-fat cheese instead of regular cheese.
- Use fat-free, low-fat, soy, or nonfat dry milk instead of whole milk.
- Use vegetable oil instead of shortening, butter, or margarine.

Reduction techniques include the following (*5,105,332*):
- Use standardized low-fat recipes.
- Use standardized low-sodium recipes.
- Use standardized low-sugar recipes.

Meat preparation techniques include the following (*5,105,332*):
- Drain fat from browned meat.
- Remove skin from poultry or use skinless poultry.
- Roast, bake, or broil meat rather than frying.
- Roast meat or poultry on a rack so fat will drain.
- Skim fat off warm broth, soup, stew, or gravy.
- Spoon solid fat from chilled meat or poultry broth.
- Trim fat from meat or use lean meat.

Vegetable preparation techniques include the following (*5,105,332*):
- Boil, mash, roast, or bake potatoes rather than frying or deep frying.

- Prepare vegetables without using butter, margarine, cheese, or creamy sauce.
- Steam, roast, grill, or bake other vegetables such as broccoli, carrots, or green beans.

Nationwide, in 2006, among schools in which school staff members had responsibility for cooking foods for students, the most commonly practiced healthy food preparation methods were using nonstick spray or pan liners instead of grease or oil; draining fat from browned meat; roasting, baking, or broiling meat rather than frying; and steaming or baking other vegetables (excluding potatoes). The least commonly practiced healthy food preparation methods were reducing sugar in recipes or using low-sugar recipes, using low-sodium canned vegetables instead of regular canned vegetables, and using cooked dry beans, canned beans, soy products, or other meat extenders instead of meat (*105*).

Schools also can use various purchasing techniques to procure healthier options while maintaining food costs. For example, local school districts can form a cooperative (co-op) to improve purchasing power with food distributors. This can increase the availability and reduce cost of healthier foods. Schools also can use USDA Foods (commodities) or ask the school district to consider creating or assigning space for a central warehouse, which allows for storage of large quantities of foods from bulk purchases and USDA Foods shipments. USDA has resources to guide schools on buying food for child nutrition programs, including the *Food Buying Guide for Child Nutrition Programs* (available at http://www.fns.usda.gov/tn/resources/foodbuyingguide.html) and *Eat Smart—Farm Fresh* (available at http://www.fns.usda.gov/cnd/guidance/farm-to-school-guidance_12-19-2005.pdf). The National Farm to School Network's website also includes resources about buying local foods (available at http://www.farmtoschool.org/publications.php?pt+othe).

Serve foods and beverages that are appealing and presented attractively. Taste tests can be used to determine which healthy options students prefer (*333–335*). When planning menus and purchasing food items that appeal to students, appearance, texture or consistency (how the food feels in the mouth and how it cuts), flavor, and service temperature (the ideal temperature for serving the food) are important (*336*). Offering various colorful fruits and vegetables with meals and snacks enhances their nutritional value and appeal. Students drink more milk when it is offered cold and in attractive packaging such as single-serving or portable plastic milk bottles (*337*). The USDA's Team Nutrition (available at http://teamnutrition.usda.gov), the School Nutrition Association (available at http://www.schoolnutrition.org), and the National Food Service Management Institute (available at http://www.nfsmi.org) offer strategies and technical assistance on serving and presenting appealing foods and beverages for school nutrition programs.

Ensure that all Foods and Beverages Sold or Served Outside of School Meal Programs Are Nutritious and Appealing

Competitive foods, which are any foods or beverages sold or served outside of the school meal program, are the principal source of the low-nutrient, energy-dense foods that students consume at school. Unlike school meals, which must meet specified nutrition standards, foods and beverages sold or provided outside of the meal program are largely exempt from federal requirements or standards. The existing federal requirement, last updated in 1985, prohibits the sale of foods of minimal nutritional value (FMNV) during meal periods in areas where reimbursable school meals are served (*338,339*). FMNV are defined as foods and beverages with <5% of the Recommended Dietary Allowances per serving for eight key nutrients; FMNV include soda, water ices, chewing gum, and certain types of candy, including gum drops, jelly beans, and candy-coated popcorn (*340,341*). The federal regulations for competitive foods prohibit the sale of FMNV. However, schools can sell these foods and beverages at other locations on the school campus during the entire school day, and other foods and beverages of low nutritional value such as chips, most candy bars, and noncarbonated, high-sugar drinks can be sold anywhere on campus, including the food service area.

The passage of the Healthy, Hunger-Free Kids Act of 2010 requires USDA to develop federal nutrition standards for competitive foods consistent with the *Dietary Guidelines for Americans* (*342*). These standards will apply to foods and beverages sold on school campus during the school day. In the last decade, a total of 39 states passed a law or policy addressing competitive foods and beverages in schools that was stronger than the current federal requirements. These state laws and policies vary in strength and breadth when compared with the IOM Nutrition Standards for Foods in School (*238,343*).

Competitive foods are offered in various school-based venues, such as à la carte in the cafeteria, vending machines, school stores and snack bars and concession stands, fundraisers on school grounds, classroom-based activities (e.g., parties and rewards or behavior-management tools), staff and parent meetings, and after-school programs (*344,345*). In 2006, 33% of elementary schools, 71% of middle schools, and 89% of high schools had a vending machine or a school store, canteen, or snack bar where students could purchase foods or beverages (*103*). The most commonly available competitive foods are high in sugar, fat, and calories, including high-fat salty snacks, high-fat baked goods, and high-calorie sugar-sweetened beverages, such as soft drinks, sports drinks, and fruit drinks

(*105,344,346*). Some progress has been made in limiting the availability of unhealthy foods in schools. For example, during 2006–2008, across 35 states, the median percentage of schools that allowed students to purchase the following items from vending machines or at the school store, canteen, or snack bar decreased: chocolate candy (from 39% to 21%), other kinds of candy (from 43% to 24%), salty snacks not low in fat (47% to 34%), soda pop (from 62% to 38%), and sports drinks (from 72% to 57%) (*347*). Consequently, offering competitive foods in vending machines at schools is associated with significantly higher BMI among middle school students (*348*). Access to sugar-sweetened beverages and low-nutrient, energy-dense foods at school significantly increases student calorie intake from sugar-sweetened beverages per school day. The third School Nutrition Dietary Assessment Study found that sugar-sweetened beverages (not including flavored milk) obtained at school contributed to an additional 29 kcal per school day for middle school students and 46 kcal per school day for high school students. Low-nutrient, energy-dense foods obtained and consumed at school contributed 86 kcal per school day for middle schools students and 111 kcal per school day for high school students. Attending schools without stores or snack bars that sell foods or beverages is estimated to significantly reduce sugar-sweetened beverage consumption by 22 kcal per school day for middle school students and 28 kcal per school day for high school students (*349*). In addition, restricting access to snack foods is associated with more frequent fruit and vegetable consumption (*350*).

In a 2001 report to Congress, USDA highlighted four major concerns about competitive foods (*351*):

1. Many competitive foods and beverages are low in nutrient density and high in fat, sugar, and calories; these products can negatively affect student diets and increase the risk for excess weight gain (*352,353*).

2. School meal programs are stigmatized when low-income students can receive free or reduced-price meals but only higher-income students can purchase competitive foods and beverages.

3. An increase in the sale of competitive foods and beverages is associated with a decrease in student participation in the reimbursable school meal program, which might affect the viability of the program (*354*).

4. Students receive inconsistent messages when they are taught about good nutrition and healthy food choices in the classroom but are surrounded by various venues offering primarily less nutritious foods.

Establish strong nutrition standards for competitive foods consistent with the IOM Nutrition Standards for Foods in Schools. Nutrition standards list criteria to help schools determine which foods and beverages should be offered on a school campus. Implementing nutrition standards can involve increasing food and beverage options, such as requiring that schools offer fruits or vegetables at all locations where other foods are available, and limiting options, such as stipulating that schools cannot sell foods with more than a specified number of calories and grams of fat per serving. State and local education agencies can pass nutrition standards that are stronger than the federal requirements limiting the sale of competitive foods.

Implementing nutrition standards can be an effective strategy to improve the nutritional quality of foods offered and purchased in the school setting (*355–357*), which might affect dietary intake (*356*). The Healthy, Hunger-Free Kids Act of 2010 requires each school district's local wellness policy to include nutritional guidelines for all foods available on each school campus that promote student health and reduce childhood obesity (*358*). Schools should implement nutrition standards that provide students with only healthy choices throughout the regular and extended school day and throughout the campus that are consistent with and reinforce positive nutrition education messages received in the classroom. Fruits, vegetables, whole grain products, and fat-free or low-fat dairy products should be offered, whereas foods that do not contain important nutrients; foods that are high in fat, added sugar, or sodium; and sugar-sweetened beverages should be eliminated or limited. Portion sizes should be reasonable for the age of the student (*35*).

IOM used a rigorous scientific review process to develop the Nutrition Standards for Foods in Schools, which provides guidance on which foods and beverages schools should offer on school campuses (*238*). The IOM standards recommend that all competitive food offerings be consistent with the *Dietary Guidelines for Americans* and, in particular, help children and adolescents meet the guidelines for consumption of fruits, vegetables, whole grains, and fat-fat or low-fat milk or milk products (*238*). The IOM standards include 13 standards for foods and beverages sold and available on campus during the school day, after-school activities, evening and community events, and on-campus fundraising. The standards address the nutritive (e.g., calories, saturated fat, sodium, and sugars) and nonnutritive components (e.g., caffeine and nonnutritive sweeteners) of foods and beverages, restrict the marketing of foods and beverages, and prohibit the use of foods and beverages as rewards or punishment. CDC created four audience-specific fact sheets about the IOM standards that can serve as a resource to support the development of strong nutrition standards for foods outside of school meal programs. These fact sheets answer common questions about the IOM standards and provide recommendations for implementation (available at http://www.cdc.gov/Healthyyouth/nutrition/standards.htm).

Schools should systematically track the financial implications of implementing strong nutrition standards. Limited data are available on the impact of changes in nutrition standards in schools on total revenue generated by sales of food and beverages (*359*). However, mounting evidence suggests that schools can maintain financial stability while offering only foods and beverages that meet strong nutrition standards (*268,360–364*). Implementing strong nutrition standards can increase school lunch participation, which financially benefits schools (*360,361,363*). Strategic promotion of healthier food and beverage choices (*355*) and lowering the price of healthier foods (e.g., fruits, vegetables, and low-fat snacks) in school cafeterias are strategies that can minimize financial risk (*272,273*). (Additional information is available at http://www.cdc.gov/healthyyouth/nutrition/pdf/financial_implications.pdf.)

Use the contracting process to improve the nutritional quality of competitive foods and beverages. Most secondary school students (67% of middle or junior high schools and 83% of high schools) attend schools that have beverage contracts (*365*). Schools that adopt strong nutrition standards for competitive foods should revise existing food and beverage contracts so that healthier options are available for students (*359*). Vending machine contracts that schools establish with food and beverage companies give the companies selling rights in return for cash and noncash benefits or incentive items such as scoreboards, cups, T-shirts, posters, and drink bottles (*365*). Schools and school districts can cancel, not sign, not renew, or negotiate contracts so that only foods and beverages that meet strong nutrition standards are available to students. For example, some schools have new districtwide vending contracts to centralize purchasing and approval of foods and beverages sold and have placed the management of new contracts under school nutrition departments to ensure better nutritional content of vending machine items (*366*). The National Policy and Legal Analysis Network to Prevent Childhood Obesity has resources to support schools in using the contracting process to improve the nutritional quality of foods and beverages sold on school property and how to negotiate favorable terms and conditions in vending contracts (available at http://www.nplanonline.org). State departments of education can support schools by providing online nutrition calculators or an updated list of products that meet nutrition standards. Schools can use these tools to ensure that products meet nutrition standards and help select products to include in a vending contract.

Market healthier foods and beverages. Schools can take advantage of marketing strategies to promote the appeal of healthier foods and beverages in various ways. Marketing healthy options might persuade students to purchase healthy foods and beverages. For example, cafeteria taste tests offer students an opportunity to taste the healthier options offered in the cafeteria (*355,367*). Taste testing provides students an opportunity to inform staff members which healthy food and beverage products they like and dislike (*268*). Strategies to promote the appeal of fruits and vegetables in schools and influence student purchases of healthy foods and beverages include (*268,368–371*)

- offering a free fruit and vegetable program;
- having students grow vegetables in a school garden;
- offering vegetables and dip on à la carte lines;
- moving fruits and vegetables to the front of the school meal serving line;
- offering sliced or wedged versions of fruits and vegetables;
- using colorful and imaginative language and images of fruits and vegetables on menus, in hallways, and in the cafeteria;
- collecting suggestions from students and families for meals and snack items that might be offered; and
- improving the lighting in the serving area and placing the salad bar near the cashier rather than away from the main serving area.

Additional strategies for low-cost changes to improve the lunch room environment are available at http://smarterlunchrooms.org.

Schools also can build partnerships to market healthy food choices to students (*372*). Strategies to present a consistent message for offering healthier foods and beverages throughout the school community include linking the cafeteria with the classroom (e.g., discussing health benefits of specific fruits and vegetables in the classroom and offering these fruits and vegetables in the cafeteria at the same time); building connections with community partners such as supermarkets, restaurants, youth-serving agencies, and local farms or farmers' organizations (e.g., hosting a school market program that works with local vendors to sell fruits and vegetables during the school day in a store managed by students); and connecting with local or regional vendor associations to partner on a healthy foods and beverages promotion campaign (e.g., partnering with the regional dairy association on a healthy milk vending program) (*368,373,374*). Schools can involve students in leading changes toward healthier competitive foods and beverages. Involving students in the decision-making process can decrease resistance to change. Students can survey and poll their peers, provide valuable input to shape policy, help plan and market changes, and promote the sustainability of healthy eating initiatives. Action for Healthy Kids' Students Taking Charge program (available at http://www.studentstakingcharge.org) and the Alliance for a Healthier Generation's empowerME@school toolkit (available at http://www.empowerme2b.org) are resources that involve students in making changes for healthier food and beverage options at school.

Use fundraising activities and student rewards that support health. Schools should incorporate fundraising activities that use only healthy foods, involve physical activity, or sell nonfood items. In 2006, nearly one in four schools held fundraiser nights at fast-food restaurants, and 54% sold baked goods that were not low in fat (*105*). Fundraising that involves selling nutritious foods and beverages (e.g., fruits, vegetables, 100% fruit juice, and low-fat or fat-free dairy products) or selling nonfood items such as wrapping paper, candles, or student artwork can support student health. One study found that policies to regulate food used for fundraising were more common in middle schools than in high schools, where the sale of foods high in fat and added sugar remained a prevalent fundraising practice (*375*). Events that engage the community in physical activity, such as runs, walks, and bicycle rides, also can be used to raise money. Other examples include basketball and golf tournaments, dance-a-thons, and car washes. In addition, as described in guideline 2, schools should use constructive classroom rewards that support student health and do not include food.

Guideline 4. Implement a Comprehensive Physical Activity Program with Quality Physical Education as the Cornerstone

A substantial percentage of recommended child and adolescent physical activity can be provided through a comprehensive school-based physical activity program. A comprehensive program includes before, during, and after-school physical activity through recess and other physical activity breaks, intramurals and physical activity clubs, interscholastic sports, walk- and bicycle-to-school initiatives, and quality physical education (*376,377*). Quality physical education serves as the cornerstone of a comprehensive program because it provides the unique opportunity for students to obtain the knowledge and skills needed to establish and maintain physically active lifestyles throughout childhood and adolescence and into adulthood. A quality physical education program: 1) meets the needs of all students, 2) is an enjoyable experience for students, 3) keeps students active for most of physical education class time, 4) teaches self-management as well as movement skills, and 5) emphasizes knowledge and skills that can be used for a lifetime (*293,378*).

Other physical activity program components (e.g., recess and intramural programs) should complement rather than take the place of physical education by serving as venues for students to explore various physical activities. Recess, classroom activity breaks, intramurals, interscholastic sports, and walking and bicycling to school can provide opportunities to practice and apply the skills taught during physical education (*293,379*) (Box 4).

Require Students in Grades K–12 To Participate in Daily Physical Education that Uses a Planned and Sequential Curriculum and Instructional Practices that Are Consistent with National or State Standards for Physical Education

Physical education can increase student participation in physical activity, increase their physical fitness (*146,147,380–383*), and enhance their knowledge and skills about why and how they should be physically active (*380,384*).

Require daily physical education for students in grades K–12. Daily physical education for grades K–12 (150 minutes per week for elementary students and 225 minutes per week for secondary students) is recommended by the National Association for Sport and Physical Education (*293,379*) and the more than 30 collaborating organizations that developed the *Health, Mental Health, and Safety Guidelines for Schools* (*215*). Daily physical education also is one of the national health objectives of *Healthy People 2020* (*10*). However, in 2006, only 4% of elementary schools, 8% of middle schools, and 2% of high schools provided daily physical education or the equivalent for the entire school year for all students in the school (*144*).

Participation in daily physical education is associated with an increased likelihood of participating regularly in moderate to vigorous intensity physical activity (*118*). Daily quality physical

BOX 4. Strategies for guideline 4: Implement a comprehensive physical activity program with quality physical education as the cornerstone

---

- Require students in grades K–12 to participate in daily physical education that uses a planned and sequential curriculum and instructional practices that are consistent with national or state standards for physical education.
- Provide a substantial percentage of each student's recommended daily amount of physical activity in physical education class.
- Use instructional strategies in physical education that enhance students' behavioral skills, confidence in their abilities, and desire to adopt and maintain a physically active lifestyle.
- Provide ample opportunities for all students to engage in physical activity outside of physical education class.
- Ensure that physical education and other physical activity programs meet the needs and interests of all students.

education provides consistent instruction in various motor skills, movement forms, self-assessment and management, physical activities, and fitness activities that are important to become physically active for a lifetime.

All students should take all required physical education courses and no substitutions, waivers, or exemptions should be permitted (*385*). Schools and school districts should not allow students to be exempted from required physical education for the following reasons: enrollment in other courses, participation in school sports, participation in other school activities, participation in community sport activities, high physical fitness competency test scores, participation in vocational training, or participation in community service activities. Exemptions and waivers deprive students of instruction time that is critical for developing motor, movement, and behavioral skills that are essential for the lifelong maintenance of a physically active lifestyle; furthermore, exemptions and waivers might send the message to students that physical education is not as important as other academic content areas and activities (*385*). Among the 84% of middle schools and 95% of high schools that required physical education in 2006, 12% of middle schools and 25% of high schools allowed students to be exempted from physical education requirements for participation in school sports. Fourteen percent of these middle schools and 20% of these high schools allowed students to be exempted from physical education for participation in school activities other than sports such as band or chorus (*144*).

Achieving the recommended 225 minutes per week for physical education can be difficult in the many secondary schools that have block schedules, which feature a fewer number of classes, and these classes last longer than those at schools with different schedules. Therefore, secondary schools with block schedules are recommended to provide 450 minutes of physical education every 10 days. Schools that do not have resources (e.g., facilities and teachers) to offer daily physical education classes can gradually add more time for physical education (i.e., increase physical education from 1 or 2 days per week to at least 3 days per week).

Implement physical education curricula consistent with national or state physical education standards. Physical education curricula provide a framework for delivering age-appropriate instruction. Written curricula should be based on an appropriate sequencing of learning activities, including the following: 1) lessons focused on motor skills, physical activity, and fitness assessments that are age and developmentally appropriate; 2) methods of teaching motor, movement, and behavioral skills that ensure basic skills lead to more advanced skills; and 3) student assessment plans to appropriately monitor and reinforce student learning. Without a physical education curriculum, documenting what should be taught, what has

been taught, and whether students are achieving learning objectives or outcomes is difficult.

School districts typically are responsible for identifying and providing schools with a physical education curriculum. However, in 2006, only 55% of school districts provided a curriculum to elementary schools; 58% provided a curriculum to middle schools; and 56% provided a curriculum to high schools (*144*).

Curricula should be based on the national standards for physical education (*293*). Based on research and consensus among physical education experts, the national standards provide the framework for identifying student performance expectations for each grade level. The national standards provide guidance for states and school districts that are developing state-level standards, instructional frameworks, and curricula. A total of 71% of states require school districts or schools to follow national or state physical education standards or guidelines, and 81% of districts require schools to do so (*144*). Among these states and districts, most require or recommend standards or guidelines based on the national standards for physical education (*144*), which describe what students should know and be able to do as a result of quality physical education.

The national standards emphasize competency in motor skills and movement patterns, movement principles and strategies, regular participation in physical activity, achievement and maintenance of health-related fitness (muscular strength and endurance, cardiorespiratory fitness, flexibility, and body composition), responsible social and personal behavior in physical activity settings, and the value of physical activity for health and enjoyment. Physical education curricula should emphasize knowledge about the physical, social, and mental health benefits of physical activity; components of health-related fitness; the recommended amounts and types of physical activity needed to promote health; the relationship between physical activity and physical fitness (*293*); principles of exercise; injury prevention; energy expenditure; and social influences on physical activity (*386*). For children, adolescents, and adults, knowledge about how to be physically active might be more important than knowledge about why physical activity is beneficial (*387,388*). Thus, physical education curricula also should include the development of safe and effective individualized physical activity plans.

In 2006, CDC released the Physical Education Curriculum Analysis Tool (PECAT) (available at http://www.cdc.gov/healthyyouth/pecat). The PECAT helps school districts conduct clear, complete, and consistent analyses of written physical education curricula based on the national physical education standards. Results from PECAT can help schools enhance an existing curriculum, develop their own curriculum, or select a published curriculum for the delivery of quality physical education in schools (*389*).

Systems and criteria have been created to identify evidence-based interventions for certain school health topics such as HIV prevention. Such criteria are based on scientific evidence of effectiveness and can help school districts and schools select and approve curricula. No comprehensive system or set of criteria specifically focused on physical education curricula exists. However, the National Cancer Institute does have a system, the Research-Tested Intervention Programs (RTIPs), which includes a scoring process for comprehensive school-based programs focused on healthy eating and physical activity. Many of the programs included within RTIPs have a physical education component, although the curricula are not extensively or separately analyzed. (Additional information available at http://rtips.cancer.gov/rtips/index.do.) In addition, the Task Force on Community Preventive Services reviewed 13 studies that focused on improving physical education through policy, curriculum, and instructional changes. After the review, the task force strongly recommended enhanced school-based physical education as an intervention strategy to increase youth physical activity (*378*).

Include protocols for student assessment in physical education. A physical education curriculum should include age-appropriate protocols for student assessment (*293,379*). Student assessment in physical education should be used to determine how well students meet national or state physical education standards, align with the content delivered through instruction, and allow teachers and schools to monitor and reinforce student learning. Assessments have many formats, including demonstration of specific skills (*390*), knowledge-based testing (*386*), out-of-school assignments that support learning and practice, assessments of progress in motor skills (*391*), and establishment of active lifestyles. The National Association for Sport and Physical Education (NASPE) has various resources on student assessments (available at http://www.aahperd.org/naspe/publications/products/pemetrics.cfm and http://www.aahperd.org/naspe/publications/products/assessment.cfm).

Schools may consider conducting fitness testing to provide feedback to students and their parents, teach students how to apply behavioral skills (e.g., self-assessment, goal-setting, decision-making, and self-management), or measure school-wide fitness levels (*392*). Fitness testing also can be used to determine student achievement of national or state physical education standards that focus on maintaining a healthy fitness level (*293*). If fitness assessments are used, students should be taught the skills needed for self-monitoring or self-testing of health-related physical fitness (*392–395*). Fitness testing should be conducted in a manner that respects and preserves the dignity of all students (e.g., results kept confidential and

tests only administered after students are aware of the testing procedures). The results of physical fitness testing should not be used to assign report card grades or be used to assess program effectiveness because the validity of these measurements might vary substantially, and overall fitness and improvements in fitness are influenced by factors (e.g., genetics and physical maturation) that are beyond the control of teachers and students (*396,397*).

Provide a Substantial Percentage of Each Student's Recommended Daily Amount of Physical Activity in Physical Education Class

Even if students participate in daily physical education, they might not always be adequately active during class. Schools should adhere to the NASPE recommendations that students engage in moderate to vigorous physical activity for at least 50% of the time they spend in physical education class, one of the most critical outcome measures in determining the quality of a physical education program (*398–400*). Several observational studies of students' physical activity levels during physical education indicated that students were not moderately to vigorously physically active for at least 50% of class time (*383,401,402*). Physical education teachers often use too much of their class time for activities related to administrative and management tasks (e.g., taking attendance and making announcements) that do not facilitate moderate to vigorous physical activity (*383,403–406*).

Implement curricular and instructional practices to increase student physical activity during physical education. After a rigorous review of physical activity intervention research, the Task Force on Community Preventive Services (available at http://www.thecommunityguide.org) recommended enhanced, school-based physical education as an effective strategy for increasing physical activity among students (*378*). Schools should adopt the enhancements to physical education recommended by the task force that include making physical education classes longer, incorporating fitness activities into physical education classes, and improving curricula and instruction. Curricular and instructional changes that increase the likelihood of keeping students active during the majority of class time include the following:
- modifying traditional game rules to make games more active (*146*)
- replacing games or activities that are inherently less active (e.g., traditional softball and kickball) with more active options (e.g., soccer)
- spending time in physical education class on aerobic activities that can easily be incorporated into students' lifestyles, such as hopping, skipping, dancing, jumping rope, and aerobic games modified to be noncompetitive and that

do not include eliminating students from the game (e.g., traditional tag and dodge ball) (*381,407,408*)

- ensuring all students have enough needed equipment such as balls and jump ropes to prevent students from waiting in lines and to allow adequate time for skill practice and participation (*382,409,410*)
- having students walk or engage in other forms of physical activity, rather than sitting or standing during roll call (*146,382,409,410*)

Use Instructional Strategies in Physical Education that Enhance Students' Behavioral Skills, Confidence in Their Abilities, and Desire To Adopt and Maintain a Physically Active Lifestyle

Incorporate instructional strategies to improve students' behavioral skills in physical education and physical activity programs. Behavioral skills such as self-assessment (e.g., assessing current levels of physical activity) and self-monitoring (e.g., tracking activity levels over time), self-management, goal-setting, and decision-making might help students establish and maintain regular involvement in physical activity (*380,384,387,411,412*). Children and adolescents who believe they have the ability to address external barriers and opportunities and lead a physically active life have more motivation for participation in physical activity (*413*). Therefore, activities or assignments that enable students to identify and address external and internal barriers and opportunities for physical activity should be integrated into physical education.

Incorporate instructional strategies in physical education to improve students' confidence in their ability to be physically active and maintain physical activity behaviors. Physical education should help students master and gain confidence in motor, movement, and behavioral skills needed to establish and maintain physically active lifestyles. The development of fundamental motor skills (e.g., running, hopping, and skipping) should be taught to elementary school students (*391*). As students move into adolescence, lifetime physical activities (e.g., walking, bicycling, tennis, and swimming) that students enjoy and succeed in are important to include in physical education lessons (*293,386,387*). To master skills and establish self-confidence in their ability, students should be taught skills that are broken down into components ranging from easy to hard (*394*). Providing students with choices during physical education class might increase students' confidence in their ability to participate in physical activity in general (*414–416*). For example, allowing students to choose the type or intensity of a specific physical activity might help increase their confidence in their ability to perform the activity in the future; they can progressively add more intensity (*412*).

Incorporate instructional strategies in physical education and physical activity programs that lead to positive attitudes and perceptions toward physical activity. Influencing students' attitudes toward and perceptions of physical activity might affect their involvement in physical activity outside of physical education class (*417,418*). Physical education should encourage students to believe that physical activity is important and enjoyable. Increasing students' self-efficacy for engaging in physical activity increases the likelihood of enjoyment and therefore the likelihood of regular participation in physical activity (*384,411*). Meeting the needs and interests of all students through various activities, emphasizing the many benefits of physical activity, and integrating opportunities to apply newly acquired skills help students develop positive attitudes toward physical activity. Other teaching practices that might increase students' participation in physical activity include enthusiastic role modeling and positive verbal reinforcement for being active (*146,383,402*).

Provide Ample Opportunities for All Students To Engage in Physical Activity Outside of Physical Education Class

The school setting can offer multiple opportunities for students to enjoy physical activity outside of physical education class and increase daily amounts of physical activity, including (*377,419*)

- recess periods for unstructured or structured play in elementary schools;
- physical activity breaks;
- after-school and lunch-time intramural and physical activity clubs;
- interscholastic sports; and
- walk- and bicycle-to-school programs.

Require daily recess. All elementary schools should follow the NASPE recommendation that at least one daily 20-minute period of recess be provided to all students (*420*). In 2006, 67% of elementary schools offered recess 5 days per week for ≥20 minutes on average in all grades (*421*).

Regularly scheduled recess periods enable children to accumulate a portion of their recommended 60 minutes of daily physical activity (*422–424*). Recess allows children to apply skills learned in physical education (e.g., motor skill development, decision-making, cooperation, conflict resolution, and negotiation) (*420,425*). However, recess should not replace physical education or be used to meet time requirements set forth in physical education policies. Participation in recess is associated with academic benefits, such as improving attentiveness, concentration, behavior, and time-on-task in the classroom (*280,281,420,426–429*).

Schools might try to facilitate increased physical activity during recess by having staff members encourage students to be active; providing students with space, facilities, equipment, and supplies that can make participation in activity appealing; using point-of-decision prompts; and providing structured, organized physical activities (e.g., four-square, active tag, or flag football) for interested students (*241,420,424,425,430–432*).

Provide physical activity breaks during the school day. Another way to increase physical activity during the school day is to incorporate activity within the classroom. Some schools offer physical activity in the classroom as part of planned lessons that teach mathematics, language arts, and other academic subjects through movement. For example, teachers might read a book aloud while students walk at a moderate pace around the room. The teacher might then ask students to identify the verbs or action words in the book by acting them out through physical activity (*433*). Such activities contribute to accumulated physical activity during the school day (*434*). Physical activity within the regular classroom also can enhance on-task classroom behavior of students (*433*) and establish a school environment that promotes regular physical activity.

Offer students opportunities to participate in intramural physical activity programs during after-school hours. Intramural physical activity programs provide additional opportunities for students to achieve their recommended daily amount of physical activity. Intramural physical activities should provide opportunities for both males and females; meet the needs of students at all levels of skills and physical abilities, particularly those who are not athletically gifted; and reflect student interest (*246*). In 2006, almost half (48%) of all schools offered intramural programs (*144*). NASPE has outlined three characteristics of quality intramural programs: 1) students have a choice of activities or participation, 2) every student is given equal opportunity to participate regardless of ability level, and 3) students have the opportunity to be involved with planning and implementing activities (*246*).

Lifetime physical activities such as walking, running, hiking, swimming, tennis, dancing, and bicycling should be included in intramural programs (*246*). Partnerships with parents and community-based organizations (e.g., health and wellness facilities such as YMCAs) might increase the availability and quality of intramural programs, as well as the time students spend being active (*118,328*). Successful program implementation can be influenced by staff training on proper program implementation (*435*) and coordination with community groups (*436*).

Offer interscholastic sports. Nationwide, 77% of middle schools and 91% of high schools offered interscholastic sports programs in 2006 (*144*); in 2009, 58% of high school students reported that they had played on one or more sports teams run by their school or community group (*78*).

School or community-based sports programs provide structured time for children and adolescents to accumulate minutes of physical activity, establish cooperative and competitive skills, and learn sport-specific and performance-based skills. Evidence indicates that participation in sports is related to higher levels of participation in overall physical activity (*437–439*). In addition, participation in sports programs has been associated with improved mental health and fewer risky health behaviors (*440,441*).

Interscholastic sports programs should provide structured, competitive opportunities for students to develop both sport-specific and behavioral skills (*260*). Although typically limited to students who are athletically gifted, interscholastic sports also provide unique opportunities for applying skills (e.g., sport-specific movements) and behaviors (e.g., self-monitoring and management) taught in physical education.

Implement and promote walk- and bicycle-to-school programs. Walking and bicycling to school has become less common among school-aged children and adolescents. As of 2005, <15% of children and adolescents walked or bicycled to and from school, compared with 41% in 1969 (*110*). Students who use physically active forms of transportation have higher overall levels of physical activity (*442–444*) and are more likely to meet physical activity recommendations (*445,446*).

Federal legislation that provides funding to states to create a Safe Routes to School initiative (*110*) has enhanced the popularity of walk- and bicycle-to-school programs. Schools making changes to the built environment (e.g., adding sidewalks and crosswalks) have experienced increases in the prevalence of students walking and bicycling to school (*447*). To support communities with developing and implementing walk- and bicycle-to-school programs, CDC has developed the KidsWalk-to-School guide (available at http://www.cdc.gov/nccdphp/dnpa/kidswalk) (*448*). The guide provides users with a step-by-step checklist, implementation tools, safety tips, and ideas to make walking to school active and exciting. The National Center for Safe Routes to School provides technical assistance and professional development to states, school districts, and schools on how to develop and implement Safe Routes to School programs (available at http://www.saferoutesinfo.org).

Ensure that Physical Education and Other Physical Activity Programs Meet the Needs and Interests of All Students

All students, regardless of sex, race/ethnicity, health status, or physical or cognitive ability or disability, should have access to physical education and other physical activity programs. Physical education and physical activity programs that overemphasize team sports and do not emphasize lifetime physical activities (e.g., walking, bicycling, and tennis) could exclude potential participants (*293,379*).

Promote and ensure inclusion of all students. Children and adolescents who are obese or who have physical or cognitive disabilities, chronic diseases (e.g., diabetes or asthma), or low fitness levels might benefit from physical education and physical activity programs to increase physical activity participation, develop motor skills, improve physical fitness, and encourage enjoyment and success (*449,450*). Nationwide, 62% of schools had students with long-term physical, medical, or cognitive disabilities. Often, students who have disabilities or chronic health conditions are discouraged from participating in physical education class and other forms of physical activity. For example, among the schools that had students with disabilities enrolled, only 59% had students with long-term disabilities participate in required physical education (*144*). Rather than excluding these children from physical education and activity programs, teachers and program leaders should modify physical education and other school- and community-based programs for these students.

Whether a student with disabilities participates in the general physical education class, works with a teaching assistant in a general physical education class, participates in a separate class with teaching assistants, or receives one-on-one instruction, appropriate modifications should be in place. Such modifications include adapting activities through 1) changes in games to increase participation by students with disabilities; 2) adaptive equipment (e.g., larger or lighter bats, balls in various sizes and textures, or lowered goals or targets) that can be used with ease; 3) adapted instructional strategies such as simplified movement patterns and modified body positions; and 4) frequent rest periods (*451*). Finally, students with disabilities should have measurable physical education goals and objectives (established by the physical education teacher or other school staff members) included in their IEP. These measurable goals and objectives enable the school or school district to ensure that students' IEP physical education goals and objectives are being met (*451*).

Guideline 5. Implement Health Education that Provides Students with the Knowledge, Attitudes, Skills, and Experiences Needed for Healthy Eating and Physical Activity

Health education supports the development of health-related knowledge, skills, and attitudes to increase the likelihood that students engage in healthy behaviors and to avoid or reduce health risks. Health education curricula and instruction should address various health topics, including healthy eating and physical activity, systematically and sequentially to ensure attainment of national and state standards and corresponding learning objectives and outcomes (*452,453*). Health education curricula should be developmentally appropriate and address physical, mental, emotional, and social dimensions of health to improve health knowledge, attitudes, skills, and behaviors (*452,453*) (Box 5).

BOX 5. Strategies for guideline 5: Implement health education that provides students with the knowledge, attitudes, skills, and experiences needed for healthy eating and physical activity

- Require health education from prekindergarten through grade 12.
- Implement a planned and sequential health education curriculum that is culturally and developmentally appropriate, addresses a clear set of behavioral outcomes that promote healthy eating and physical activity, and is based on national standards.
- Use curricula that are consistent with scientific evidence of effectiveness in helping students improve healthy eating and physical activity behaviors.
- Use classroom instructional methods and strategies that are interactive, engage all students, and are relevant to their daily lives and experiences.

Require Health Education from Prekindergarten Through Grade 12

Health education is integral to the primary mission of schools, providing students with the knowledge and skills they need to become successful learners and healthy adults. In 2002, the Joint Committee on Health Education Terminology defined health education as "the development, delivery, and evaluation of planned, sequential, and developmentally appropriate instruction, learning experiences, and other activities designed to protect, promote, and enhance the health literacy, attitudes, skills, and well-being of students, prekindergarten through grade 12" (*454*). Health education is a fundamental part of an overall school health program. Increasing the number of schools that require health education and teach ways to prevent important health problems, such as those resulting from poor dietary behaviors and lack of physical activity, are national health objectives (objective EMC 4) (*10*).

Most states and districts require, but devote few hours to, health education and instruction on nutrition and physical activity. Nationwide in 2006, the median number of hours of required instruction on nutrition was 3.4 hours for elementary schools, 4.2 hours for middle schools, and 5.9 for high schools. The median number of hours of required instruction on physical activity was 2.4 hours for elementary schools, 3.1 hours for middle schools, and 4.5 for high schools (*455*). Schools also require less health education as students progress through school. Almost two thirds (61%) of all schools required health instruction in at least one specific grade, but 34% of schools with 9th-grade students required it in 9th grade, 25% in 10th grade, 12% in 11th grade, and 9% in 12th grade (*455*).

Nutrition and physical activity topics also can be integrated into other academic disciplines to complement comprehensive health education and physical education programs (*456,457*). Examples might include biology lessons on energy balance (*458*) and the physics of body movement, math lessons on nutrient analysis, family and consumer science courses on cooking skills, and language arts lessons analyzing food advertisements (*459*). Integration of health topics throughout the school curriculum should not replace health education as a course in school; a comprehensive health education curriculum is necessary to enable students to achieve the national and state standards for health education. Schools that rely on integration into other academic areas as the sole means of providing health education might provide less instructional time for health and cover fewer topics than when health education is a separate course.

Implement a Planned and Sequential Health Education Curriculum that Is Culturally and Developmentally Appropriate, Addresses a Clear Set of Behavioral Outcomes that Promote Healthy Eating and Physical Activity, and Is Based on National Standards

Implement a planned and sequential curriculum that is culturally and developmentally appropriate. Health education curricula should include (*453*)

- clearly articulated learning outcomes or learning objectives;
- a planned progression of developmentally and culturally appropriate lessons or learning experiences that lead to achieving these objectives;
- continuity between lessons or learning experiences that clearly reinforce the adoption and maintenance of specific health-enhancing behaviors;
- accompanying content or materials that correspond with the sequence of learning events and help teachers and students meet the learning objectives;
- consideration of cultural heritage, family attitudes and customs, and differences in physical activity and diet of students when designing lesson plans; and

- assessment strategies to determine whether students have achieved the desired learning objectives.

Health education should incorporate student assessment strategies that enable students to demonstrate their understanding of primary health concepts and apply health-related skills to real-life situations. Quality health education assessment protocols include criteria for examining student work (such as a rubric) and incorporate multiple measures over time (*453,460,461*).

A student assessment should help improve and inform teaching practices and promote learning (*453,462–464*), use multiple sources of information, and provide fair, valid, and reliable information (*453,465*). The choice of specific assessment methods should be determined by the nature of the learning outcomes being assessed, the purpose of the assessments, and the grade level of the students (*466*). Assessments that are performance based (rather than based on recall and recognition) enable students to apply knowledge and skills and are well-suited to learning skills such as effective decision-making and interpersonal communication (*453,462,467*). Performance-based assessments are designed to measure a student's knowledge, ability, skill, and attitude consistently, emphasizing methods other than standardized achievement tests, particularly those using multiple-choice formats (*453,465,468,469*). Performance-based assessments typically include performance tasks, exhibitions, demonstrations, written or oral responses, journals, and portfolios (*465,469*). Examples include photo essays, skits, infomercials, public service announcements, and letters to the editor.

Implement a curriculum that addresses a clear set of behavioral outcomes that promote healthy eating and physical activity. Health education that incorporates the topics of healthy eating and physical activity has been shown to improve student dietary behaviors (*148,467,470–472*) and physical activity participation levels (*148,217*); reduce sedentary behaviors (*159,457,473*); and improve serum cholesterol levels (*474–476*), blood pressure (*474,477*), and BMI (*457,459,474,477*). School-based type 2 diabetes prevention programs with health education components have resulted in increased knowledge about the disease (*478,479*) and improvements in student blood glucose levels for diverse groups of students at high risk for the disease (*480–482*).

Nutrition education should be part of a comprehensive school health education curriculum. As a result of participation in a K–12 health education curriculum that includes nutrition, students should have the knowledge and skills to do the following (*199,200,462,483*):

- Eat a variety of whole grain products, fruits and vegetables, and nonfat or low-fat milk or equivalent milk products every day.

- Eat the appropriate amounts from each food group every day.
- Choose foods that provide ample amounts of vitamins and minerals.
- Eat the appropriate amounts of high-fiber foods.
- Drink plenty of water.
- Limit foods and beverages high in added sugar.
- Limit the intake of fat, avoiding foods with saturated and trans fats.
- Eat breakfast every day.
- Eat healthy snacks.
- Eat healthy food when dining out.
- Prepare food in healthy ways.
- Balance caloric intake with caloric expenditure.
- Follow a plan for healthy weight management.
- Support others to eat healthy.

Health education curricula should reinforce the information taught in physical education classes and provide opportunities for students to apply physical activity knowledge and skills. As a result of participation in a K–12 health education curriculum that includes physical activity, students should have the knowledge and skills to be able to do the following (147,462):

- Engage in moderate to vigorous physical activity for at least 60 minutes every day.
- Regularly engage in physical activities that enhance cardiorespiratory endurance, flexibility, muscle endurance, and muscle strength.
- Engage in warm-up and cool-down activities before and after exercise.
- Drink plenty of water before, during, and after physical activity.
- Follow a physical activity plan for healthy weight management.
- Avoid injury during physical activity.
- Support others to be physically active.

Health education should foster positive attitudes toward being a physically active person by emphasizing the benefits and enjoyment of physical activity, supporting students who are physically active, and incorporating self-management techniques (e.g., assessing personal physical activity level and setting goals to be more active) into lessons (484).

Skill-based health education also should include lessons on limiting sedentary screen time (e.g., television, video games, and computer usage). Studies have found that such lessons can reduce television viewing and other screen and media time among students and demonstrate promise in preventing childhood obesity (159,457,473). The Task Force on Community Preventive Services conducted a rigorous review of research and recommended behavioral interventions to reduce screen time among preschool children and school-aged children and adolescents. The seven interventions included in the review

focused on establishing classes for building skills, tips, setting goals, and reinforcement techniques, and parent or family support through schools or other organizations providing information on environmental strategies to reduce exposure to and use of televisions, computers, and video games. (Additional details about the review are available at http://www.thecommunityguide.org/obesity/behavioral.html.) Finally, health education curricula should focus on building student skills (e.g., self-monitoring, setting goals, and decision-making) to help decrease television viewing, decrease consumption of high-fat food, increase fruit and vegetable intake, and increase physical activity (457,473).

Implement health education curricula that are consistent with the National Health Education Standards. The National Health Education Standards and performance indicators outline the health-related concepts, skills, and healthy beliefs, values, and norms students need for healthy behaviors (453). These standards provide a foundation for selecting or developing curricular and instructional materials, delivering instruction, and assessing student knowledge, attitudes, skills, and behaviors. Many state boards of education, state departments of education, and local school boards have adopted their own state or local health education standards using the National Health Education Standards as a guide. In 2006, most (72%) states required or encouraged districts or schools to follow health education standards or guidelines based specifically on the national standards, and most districts (66%) required or encouraged the same for schools (455). A national health objective strives to increase the proportion of elementary, middle, and senior high schools that have health education goals or objectives that address the knowledge and skills in the National Health Education Standards (high school, middle school, and elementary school) (objective ECBP 3) (10).

The National Health Education Standards emphasize the development of skills and specify that, as a result of health education, students should be able to 1) understand concepts related to health promotion and disease prevention; 2) analyze the influence of family, peers, culture, media, technology, and other factors on health behaviors; 3) access valid information, products, and services to enhance health; 4) use interpersonal communication skills to enhance health and avoid or reduce health risks; 5) use decision-making skills to enhance health; 6) use goal-setting skills to enhance health; 7) practice health-enhancing behaviors and avoid or reduce health risks; and 8) advocate for personal, family, and community health (453).

CDC's Health Education Curriculum Analysis Tool (HECAT) helps school districts conduct clear, complete, and consistent analyses of written health education curricula based on the National Health Education Standards and research-based characteristics of effectiveness. HECAT addresses a wide range of health topics, including modules on healthy eating and physical activity. Results from HECAT can help schools enhance an existing curriculum, develop their own curriculum, or select a published curriculum that will deliver quality health education (462). The tool is available online at http://www.cdc.gov/HealthyYouth/hecat.

Use Curricula that Are Consistent with Scientific Evidence of Effectiveness in Helping Students Improve Healthy Eating and Physical Activity Behaviors

Health education curricula, regardless of the topic, should reflect the research that emphasizes teaching functional health information (essential concepts), shaping personal values that support healthy behaviors, shaping group norms that value a healthy lifestyle, and developing essential health skills necessary to adopt and maintain health-enhancing behaviors. Similar to physical education, most of the school-based programs included in RTIPs have a health education component; however, the curricula are not extensively or separately analyzed (additional information available at http://rtips.cancer.gov/rtips/index.do). Health education curricula and materials should be based on theories of behavior change and have the following characteristics (453):

- focus on clear health goals and specific behavioral outcomes
- be research-based and theory-driven
- address individual values and group norms that support health-enhancing behaviors
- focus on increasing the personal perception of risk and harmfulness of engaging in specific health risk behaviors as well as reinforcing protective factors
- address social pressures and influences
- build personal competence, social competence, and increase confidence in skills
- provide functional health knowledge that is basic and accurate and directly contributes to health-promoting decisions and behaviors
- use strategies designed to personalize information and engage students
- provide age-appropriate and developmentally appropriate information, learning strategies, teaching methods, and materials
- incorporate learning strategies, teaching methods, and materials that are culturally inclusive
- provide adequate time for instruction and learning
- provide opportunities to reinforce skills and positive health behaviors
- provide opportunities to make positive connections with influential others

- include teacher information and plans for professional development that enhance effectiveness of instruction and student learning

Use Classroom Instructional Methods and Strategies that Are Interactive, Engage All Students, and Are Relevant to Their Daily Lives and Experiences

Health education instruction should include the use of active learning strategies that encourage student participation and help develop the concepts, attitudes, and skills needed to make healthy eating choices and be physically active from childhood through adulthood (485). Interactive lessons that include demonstration, modeling, rehearsal, and feedback are more likely to result in positive behavioral changes than a traditional didactic approach (148,482,486,487). The use of goal-setting skills also can be integrated into health education to help students identify personal goals for dietary and physical activity behaviors (488). Adequate professional development should be offered to teachers because these active learning strategies may be unfamiliar to some (182).

Use interactive learning strategies. Students are more likely to adopt healthy eating and physical activity behaviors when

- they learn about these behaviors through enjoyable, participatory activities rather than through lectures (230,488–490);
- lessons emphasize the positive, appealing aspects of physical activity and healthy eating patterns rather than the negative consequences and present the benefits in the context of what is already important to students (491–494); and
- they have repeated opportunities to practice physical activity and healthy eating behaviors that are relevant to their daily lives (485,488,489,495,496).

Use methods and strategies that are developmentally appropriate. Educational strategies should match the different stages of students' cognitive development. For example, nutrition education for younger children should focus on concrete experiences, such as increasing exposure to many healthy foods and building skills in choosing healthy foods (230,490,497). By middle school, students can understand and act on the connection between physical activity, healthy eating behaviors, and their overall health as well as the role these behaviors play in preventing chronic diseases (453,491).

Developmentally appropriate strategies for adolescents include skill development (such as learning a dance or preparing a certain fruit), self-monitoring (such as a diary of physically active and sedentary behaviors or tracking fruit and vegetable consumption), and promotion of regular physical activity and healthy eating (498). Health education for middle and high school students should focus on self-assessment and setting personal goals (*498,499*). Lessons for older students should emphasize personal responsibility for making healthy and positive choices, decision-making skills for healthy eating and physical activity, analysis of dietary and physical activity behaviors and their influence on chronic disease risk, resisting negative social pressures, and advocating for individual, family, and community health (*500–502*). HECAT provides concepts and skill examples deemed appropriate for various grade groups (i.e., grades prekinderten–2, 3–5, 6–8, and 9–12).

Integrate computer-based instruction into health education. Computer-based instruction on physical activity and healthy eating offers opportunities for self-paced health education (*485,495,503,504*). Interactive computer programs can help students learn and assess their own physical activity and healthy eating skills (*505–507*). For example, students can track via computer their daily physical activity for a week and receive a report on how many days they met the physical activity guidelines. Students also can be exposed to interactive computer programs that enable them to track the foods they have eaten over a given period and receive a nutritional analysis.

Guideline 6. Provide Students with Health, Mental Health, and Social Services to Address Healthy Eating, Physical Activity, and Related Chronic Disease Prevention

Schools are responsible for the physical health, mental health, and safety of students during the school day (*215*). School health, mental health, and social services staff members can

- teach students the skills they need to live a healthy life;
- identify risky student behaviors and intervene when needed;
- identify and resolve health-care needs that affect educational achievement;
- provide case management for health and mental health issues;
- address behavioral and psychological problems;
- link students and families to community health resources; and
- provide overall leadership for school health programs, including those designed to promote physical activity and healthy eating.

School health, mental health, and social services are accessible to students who have special needs or chronic health conditions and those who do not have health insurance or might not make regular visits to a health-care provider. Qualified professionals such as nurses, physicians, dentists, health educators, and other allied health personnel provide school health services. Professionals such as certified school counselors, psychologists, social workers, and, occasionally, psychiatrists provide mental health and social services (*508*). Schools can refer students for additional care to community agencies, organizations, or health-care providers not on the school property or to school-based health centers.

School nurses can play a critical role in coordinating student health-care services at the school. When necessary, they coordinate with community health-care providers or school-based health centers providing care to students (*509*). A national health objective aims to increase the proportion of the U.S. schools that have a nurse-student ratio of at least 1:750 well children (objective ECBP 5) (*10*). Certain schools might need a higher nurse-student ratio for students who require daily professional nursing services or students with complex health needs (*509*). In 2006, 45% of all schools had a nurse-student ratio of at least 1:750; 36% of all schools had a full-time school nurse (*510*).

School nurses should have a minimum of a bachelor's degree in nursing. A certification in the specialty of school nursing is preferred, with a current state license as a registered nurse to be able to serve both as a full-time health-care provider and health educator (*509,511,512*). School nurses have the knowledge and expertise to address a range of services that includes promotion of healthy eating, physical activity, and weight management (*513*). Schools also need access to a consulting physician to provide services such as school-based standing orders, consultations and supplementary training for staff members, recommendations for families, review of school health and health services policies and procedures, and communication with and referrals to physicians or other health-care providers (*182,215,509*). To address mental health concerns, schools might link students to school-based health centers or community-based services or employ mental health and social services staff members.

Because of the range of activities that require the involvement of various professionals, staff members should work collaboratively to coordinate student care and school health, mental health, and social services both within and outside of the school setting (*215,509,514–517*). The goal of staff collaboration within the school setting should be to provide consistent messages about health behaviors to all students; delegate case management to the staff member with the most appropriate training, competency, and licensure for a particular health issue (*215*); and coordinate care among health, mental health, and social services staff members when students have physical health conditions that might coexist with mental health problems (Box 6).

BOX 6. Strategies for guideline 6: Provide students with health, mental health, and social services to address healthy eating, physical activity, and related chronic disease prevention

- Assess student needs related to physical activity, nutrition, and obesity, and provide counseling and other services to meet those needs.
- Ensure students have access to needed health, mental health, and social services.
- Provide leadership in advocacy and coordination of effective school physical activity and nutrition policies and practices.

Assess Student Needs Related to Physical Activity, Nutrition, and Obesity, and Provide Counseling and Other Services To Meet Those Needs

Identification, follow-up, and treatment of health and mental health conditions related to diet, physical activity, and weight are important for student health (182,518). School health, mental health, and social services staff members should collaborate with community health-care providers to increase student access to care, coordinate care, and promote evidence-based physical activity and healthy eating initiatives (215). Schools should link students to appropriate services within the local medical community that are staffed by employees with appropriate training and are accessible to all students, including those with low family incomes or without insurance (215). Schools also should identify and link students and their families to community-based health promotion programs that encourage physical activity and healthy eating.

Assess eating and physical activity behaviors of students. School nurses, together with other health, mental health and social services staff members, can assess the healthy eating and physical activity behaviors of students during routine interactions. Information about the number of students in the school who meet diet, physical activity, and weight status recommendations can be used to guide program planning and policy advocacy efforts. Assessment also enables staff members to identify students in need of counseling and referral services. Some student assessment results might reveal signs and symptoms of health risks that require urgent attention, such as hypertension, hunger, use of illegal performance-enhancing drugs, or disordered eating. All school staff members may be given guidance on how to recognize early signs of these risk behaviors and confidentially refer students with diet, physical activity, or mental health concerns to health, mental health, and social services staff members. Students with signs of serious conditions or health risk behaviors should be referred to a primary health-care provider (519).

Following are some of the topics that a health practitioner can address during a rapid dietary assessment. Evidence indicates that these behaviors are associated with energy intake and can be a focus of change if needed (37,38,520):

- frequency of eating fast food or outside the home in restaurants
- usual daily intake of sugar-sweetened beverages and 100% fruit juice
- typical portion sizes
- frequency of eating breakfast
- usual daily intake of foods that are high in energy density
- usual intake of fruits and vegetables
- meal frequency and snacking patterns

Staff members should also refer to the *Dietary Guidelines for Americans* for current recommendations for dietary intakes for children and adolescents (5).

Following are some topics that a health practitioner can address during a rapid physical activity assessment (37,38,520):

- amount of daily physical activity participation (e.g., whether student is physically active for ≥60 minutes per day through free play, time spent outside, physical education, and involvement in organized activities such as school or community recreation programs)
- number of hours per day of television, movies, video game, and computer use (e.g., whether student is viewing >1–2 hours of quality programming per day)
- presence of a television or a computer in student's bedroom
- participation in physical education classes
- amount of physically active discretionary activities, such as walking or bicycling to school, taking stairs, or doing chores

Staff members also should refer to the 2008 *Physical Activity Guidelines for Americans* (9), the CDC Youth Physical Activity Guidelines Toolkit (available at http://www.cdc.gov/healthyyouth/physicalactivity/guidelines.htm), and AAP policy guidance on screen time (160).

Staff members also might refer to the National Association of School Nurses' SCOPE (School Nurse Childhood Obesity Prevention Education) manual (521) or the AAP's Pediatric Obesity Clinical Decision Support Chart (522). The questions should be age appropriate; students aged <10 years might not be able to answer questions as reliably as older students. Obtaining a more accurate assessment of younger students might require posing questions to parents or caregivers (520).

Schools initiating BMI measurement programs should implement safeguards. In many schools, nurses measure students' height and weight and use the results to determine their BMI status. Data on the percentage of students who are obese and overweight in a school or school district can be useful for program planning, policy advocacy efforts, and evaluation. Some schools send BMI results home to students' families, along with guidance on improving student physical activity and nutrition behaviors. This process is often called BMI screening. BMI information can help correct parent and student misperceptions about weight status and might motivate families to seek medical care and make healthy lifestyle changes. However, there is not enough evidence to recommend for or against BMI screening programs in schools (518). Research studies have not yet fully assessed the usefulness of school-based BMI screening in preventing and reducing obesity among students; the impact of BMI screening on weight-related knowledge, attitudes, and the behaviors of students and their families; or of any potential harm that might result from such screening (e.g., stigmatizing students or encouraging harmful weight loss practices) (518). In 2007, an expert panel recommended that BMI should be calculated and plotted at least annually at all well-child visits at the primary health-care provider (38). Schools that make the decision to conduct BMI screening should implement safeguards to ensure respect for students' privacy and confidentiality, protect students from potential harm, and increase the likelihood that the program will have a positive impact on promoting a healthy weight. Schools should ensure that appropriate follow-up diagnosis and care are available to students at a community health-care provider. Essential safeguards for and more detailed information about school-based BMI measurement programs are described in CDC's document, *Body Mass Index Measurement in Schools* (available at http://www.cdc.gov/healthyyouth/obesity/bmi/pdf/BMI_execsumm.pdf) (518).

Counsel students on how to achieve healthy eating and physical activity recommendations. Counseling can begin with motivational interviewing, a nonjudgmental, empathetic, and encouraging approach that allows students to express positive or negative feelings toward healthy eating and physical activity and identify their own reasons and plans for improvement. Motivational interviewing involves staff members asking, informing, advising, and listening about healthy eating and physical activity behaviors. Staff members who provide counseling should have the appropriate training necessary to counsel students about eating healthfully and being active (520). Student assessment results will guide the counseling sessions, and staff members can ask students to identify the behavior they might be interested in changing or that might be easiest to change (37,520). Staff members can further assess students' readiness and motivation to change by asking how important it is to them and how confident they feel about their ability to change. Counseling that involves students' families might have a greater impact on the environmental influences that shape students' diet and physical activity behaviors away from school (37).

Subsequent to assessment and motivational interviewing, staff members can use behavioral strategies, such as goal-setting, positive reinforcement, and self-monitoring, to facilitate changes in students' health behaviors (520). Goal-setting should be a process, incrementally moving toward the desired outcomes (e.g., increase physical activity by 10% per week) (520,523). Staff members should schedule follow-up sessions to assess students' progress toward their goals (520).

Students who are already active and have healthy diets should be encouraged to continue these behaviors. Emphasizing the benefits of healthy eating and regular physical activity and encouraging students to be role models for their peers are ways to reinforce these behaviors (215,498,524).

Students with eating disorders, who are binge eating, or who have other weight concerns might need more specific mental health and social services (519). Obese students, for example, are at increased risk for being teased, bullied, or socially isolated and having low self-esteem and depression (35,282,525–529). Students with weight concerns are at increased risk for unhealthy dieting behaviors (530,531). In addition, students with extreme perceptions of body size (e.g., perceive themselves as very overweight) are at increased risk for suicide ideation and suicide attempts (532). Health, mental health, and social services staff members should be prepared to promote positive body image and body satisfaction; help students overcome barriers to healthy eating and physical activity; help students find social support, cope with teasing, set goals, and make decisions; and refer students who might require primary medical care (518). All staff members should be aware of early signs and symptoms of mental health problems that might become evident during physical activity, dietary, and weight assessments (519).

Manage the physical activity and nutritional needs of students with chronic health conditions. Diet and physical activity are critical to the management of many chronic health conditions, such as asthma, diabetes, obesity, and food allergies. Health, mental health, and social services staff members should be attentive to students with these conditions to ensure they are meeting healthy eating and activity recommendations (533–535). Health services staff members, in partnership with medical providers and families, play a key role in developing and coordinating the implementation of individualized health plans established for students with chronic health conditions (509,533,534,536,537) and encouraging them to participate fully in structured and unstructured physical activity, regardless of ability, unless medically contraindicated. Health, mental health, and social services staff members can collaborate with students' families and health-care providers to maximize student participation, provide modified activities when appropriate, and eliminate barriers to student participation.

Families and health-care providers should notify schools about dietary restrictions or modifications and schedules for meals and snacks related to the condition (*519*). Health, mental health, and social services staff members can request written permission from families to exchange confidential health information with students' health-care providers (*515*). Trained school health staff members can collaborate with students' primary health-care providers to ensure monitoring of vital signs and compliance with treatment program and to address students' health issues in a confidential and sensitive manner (*519*). These efforts ensure that students who require ongoing management for chronic health conditions will receive continuous care and monitoring at school. This network is important to facilitate quick notification to all parties when a change is observed in the students' health status or when there is a revision to the health management plan (*538*).

If a student has a medical provider–prescribed weight management plan, then health, mental health, and social services staff members can communicate with the student's health-care provider to discuss their role in monitoring implementation and assisting the student with compliance. Unless specified otherwise, the goal of the weight management strategy should be weight maintenance versus weight loss. To ensure appropriate and safe oversight, the health, mental health, and social services staff member coordinating care with the student's health-care provider needs to have training in pediatric weight management or behavioral counseling (*539*). The *Expert Committee Recommendations Regarding the Prevention, Assessment, and Treatment of Child and Adolescent Overweight and Obesity* include detailed guidance on assessment, counseling, and management for health-care workers providing care for overweight and obese young persons (*37,38,520,539*).

Ensure Students Have Access to Needed Health, Mental Health, and Social Services

Health, mental health, and social services staff members serve as liaisons between school staff members, students, families, community programs, and health-care providers (*515*). Community resources can address health, mental health, and social service gaps that the school might not have the resources or expertise to address adequately. In addition, this collaborative approach keeps the community informed about school-based healthy eating and physical activity initiatives and keeps school staff members aware of community-based services (*520*). Health, mental health, and social services staff members should seek out partnerships and serve on community health coalitions (*515*). Coordination of services might increase student and family participation in community-based healthy eating, physical activity, and obesity prevention programs (*540–542*).

Refer students to community-based health-care providers and healthy eating and physical activity services. School health personnel should establish systematic processes and criteria for referring students to external primary health-care providers (*215*). Students with signs of disordered eating or diet-related health conditions (e.g., sudden weight loss, eating disorders, or obesity) should be referred to a primary health-care provider for diagnosis and, if needed, establishment of management or treatment plans. For example, students classified as obese or overweight after BMI screening require further medical examination to determine whether the student in fact has excess body fat or other conditions related to obesity (e.g., diabetes or prediabetes, high blood cholesterol and triglyceride levels, or early pubertal maturation) (*543–545*).

Health, mental health, and social services staff members play an important role in developing and marketing a referral system for students and families (*215,498,513,535*). To establish a referral system, health, mental health, and social services staff members should identify health-care services and school- or community-based programs that encourage healthy eating and physical activity and address obesity and eating disorders. These services include school-linked health clinics, local health departments, universities, medical schools, outside health-care providers (e.g., private physicians and dentists, hospitals, psychologists and other mental health workers, pediatric weight management clinics, community health clinics, and managed care organizations), and community-based nutrition and physical activity providers and services (e.g., dieticians, recreational programs, and cooking classes).

The list of referral services should be based on the health needs of the student population, barriers to health care in the community, past student use of community services, and current community culture. Health, mental health, and social services staff members can assess which services are available at the school and which require outside referral (*182*). The list should include services that are accessible to all students, including those with low family incomes or without health insurance or transportation. If feasible, arrangements can be made to bring community-based services to the school. With a comprehensive referral system in place, health, mental health, and social services staff members are able to respond to requests from families seeking guidance and increase access to care among students (*546*).

Provide Leadership in Advocacy and Coordination of Effective School Physical Activity and Nutrition Policies and Practices

Health, mental health, and social services staff members can take an active role in implementing coordinated school health practices and be highly involved in the school health council

(513,515). Staff members can work through the school health council to establish policies and practices that promote the school health agenda.

In addition to providing care directly to students, school nurses can coordinate school health, mental health, and social services staff member efforts to advocate for a healthy school environment; increase student and staff member knowledge and promote healthy behaviors through health education; lead efforts to assess, develop, and evaluate health policies, practices, and programs; and serve as a liaison between teachers and families regarding student health needs (515,519,542,547–549).

Advocate on behalf of students to create a healthy, safe, and supportive school environment that allows students to make healthy dietary and physical activity choices both in and out of school. School health advocacy raises awareness about the importance of health behaviors and can increase school and community support for instruction, programs, policies, and environmental changes that support healthy eating and physical activity (550). Effective advocacy requires collaboration within the school setting and in the broader community. Health, mental health, and social services staff members are ideally situated to engage community health-care providers and organizations in supporting healthy eating and physical activity policies and practices within schools (540,541,551).

Health, mental health, and social services staff members can advocate for schools to develop strong policies and practices that help students achieve healthy eating and physical activity recommendations (515,520,552–554). Advocacy efforts should promote a safe and supportive environment for all students, regardless of athletic ability, weight status, special needs, or chronic health condition (515). For example, they can support adoption of a universal bullying prevention program to address disrespectful behavior and prevent bullying of students with chronic health conditions or weight issues and all other students (518). Health, mental health, and social services staff members can work with physical education and health education teachers, nutrition service staff members, principals, and other school staff members to establish a healthy environment and consistently promote healthy eating and physical activity messages and activities throughout the school setting (542,550,555).

Guideline 7. Partner with Families and Community Members in the Development and Implementation of Healthy Eating and Physical Activity Policies, Practices, and Programs

Families and community members (including community organizations) contribute to the academic success of students and are key stakeholders in healthy eating and physical activity policies and practices in schools (556–558). Partnerships among schools, families, and community members can enhance student learning, promote consistent messages about healthy behaviors, increase resources, and engage, guide, and motivate students to eat healthfully and be active (557,559). These three sectors of society influence the growth and development of children and adolescents and share the responsibility for nurturing them into healthy and productive adults (557,559).

Families shape the context of children's everyday social and physical environments; they control the availability of food and influence eating and activity practices (560–562). Although evaluations of the effects of family involvement in school and community-based health interventions have been inconclusive (largely because of variability in study design and inadequate family participation) (334,472,479,563–577), certain findings are worth noting. Family involvement in health can increase their children's knowledge and attitudes about healthy lifestyles (569), influence behavior change (570,575,576,578–581), and provide social support for being healthy (573). Studies that have assessed strategies to prevent and treat childhood obesity or promote physical activity and healthy eating have demonstrated more success when focusing on both the family and the child rather than the child alone (571,578,579,582).

Community partners, including individual persons, agencies, and organizations, can offer multiple resources for healthy eating and physical activity initiatives at schools (e.g., sharing health services) (556,559), provide funding, provide guidance on specific health topics, and provide volunteer support (447,559,583,584). Partners might include businesses, health departments, community health educators, health-care providers, health-care organizations, parks and recreation departments, universities and educational institutions, transportation authorities and other government agencies, faith-based organizations, senior citizen organizations, cultural institutions, local foundations, national service and volunteer organizations, local chefs, and other community volunteers (556).

To develop successful and meaningful partnerships, all partners involved should demonstrate a commitment to student health and communicate intent and expectations about their level of involvement and respective roles in making decisions. Schools should provide a respectful and welcoming climate to families and outside organizations, and the school principal should fully support outside involvement (*556*) (Box 7).

BOX 7. Strategies for guideline 7: Partner with families and community members in the development and implementation of healthy eating and physical activity policies, practices, and programs

- Encourage communication among schools, families, and community members to promote adoption of healthy eating and physical activity behaviors among students.
- Involve families and community members on the school health council.
- Develop and implement strategies for motivating families to participate in school-based programs and activities that promote healthy eating and physical activity.
- Access community resources to help provide healthy eating and physical activity opportunities for students.
- Demonstrate cultural awareness in healthy eating and physical activity practices throughout the school.

Encourage Communication Among Schools, Families, and Community Members to Promote Adoption of Healthy Eating and Physical Activity Behaviors Among Students

Communicate frequently and use various dissemination methods. Schools should communicate with families and community members frequently to emphasize that they are a valuable asset in student learning, health, and well-being (*556,585*). Schools that communicate with families and community members about healthy eating and physical activity initiatives create a greater understanding of school activities, which might increase support and participation in school policies and practices from students and their families (*188,557*). Lines of communication should be open for feedback from families and other community members (*586,587*). Schools can work with families and community members to design needs assessments to gather information on the types of communication that families and community members would like to receive and identify resources offered within the community (*588*). Examples of topics that schools

might address with families and community members include the following:

- school healthy eating and physical activity policies (e.g., types of food allowed at school celebrations and the length of recess provided to students)
- how to provide input on policies, curricula, and programs that are being considered for adoption
- how to participate in the school health council
- nutrition and physical activity instruction in health education
- physical education instruction, including student fitness and physical activity assessment results
- opportunities for physical activity in the school (e.g., physical activity clubs, intramural sports, and interscholastic athletics)
- how to access school physical activity facilities after school hours
- what is being offered by the school nutrition services program (e.g., school breakfast program, school lunch program, menus for school meals, and nutrient analysis of school meals)
- strategies for healthy cooking at home
- school events related to physical activity and healthy eating (e.g., open houses, athletic events, and cooking workshops)
- tips on how to be physically active with children
- community resources on physical activity (e.g., parks and recreation departments), healthy eating (e.g., cooking classes, and food banks), and weight management
- opportunities to volunteer and be involved

Informational or promotional flyers, newsletters, telephone calls, conversations at school, communication via e-mail or websites, and media coverage can be used for communication with families and community members (*587,589,590*). Local media outlets provide an opportunity to disseminate school messages and remind families and community members to engage in healthy behaviors (*589,590*).

Involve Families and Community Members on the School Health Council

To participate in planning of and decision-making about school health policies and practices, families and community members should be members of the school health council. All groups invested in school health, including families and community members, and those who will be affected by policies or programs should have representation on the school health council (*194,586,591,592*). In 2006, among the 73% of school districts that had a district school health council, 89% included community members, 76% included families of students, 51% included local health-care providers, 50% included representatives from the local health department, 40%

included representatives from local social service agencies, and 26% included representatives from local health organizations (e.g., the local Red Cross chapter) (593).

The school health council should identify strategies for establishing partnerships with families and community members. The school health action plan should include goals that specifically address establishing partnerships with families and community members. To help inform the action plan, the school health council can assess the status of family and community partnerships at their school through formal questionnaires, telephone interviews, surveys, or the CDC School Health Index (199,200,556).

Families and community members should be invited to provide input on the planning and implementation of healthy eating and physical activity policies, programs, and practices. Their input will help create partnerships that appropriately blend into the community's culture, resulting in greater awareness and buy-in from students and families (557,584,586,587,591,594). Persons already active in work groups, projects, or campaigns (e.g., parent-teacher associations [PTAs]) might help recruit other interested participants through announcements, telephone trees, and reminders when families are at the school (585). Families and community members can identify potential challenges to implementation of policies, programs, and practices (588), as well as identify community supporters such as cultural or political leaders critical to the success of the initiative (589,592,594).

Develop and Implement Strategies for Motivating Families To Participate in School-Based Programs and Activities that Promote Healthy Eating and Physical Activity

In 2006, 56% of required health education classes and 31% of physical education courses incorporated homework or projects that involved family members (593). Schools and districts can provide professional development instruction for teachers on engaging families in student learning and school health program activities. In 2006, only 33% of required physical education classes or courses and 41% of required health education classes or courses had a teacher who had received instruction in the past 2 years on encouraging family and community involvement (593).

Formats for involving families include family homework assignments, healthy eating and physical activity newsletters (334,472,479,564,566,567,569–572), family nights focused on health promotion (564,572,574,577), and Internet-based programs (563). However, to have an effect on children's health knowledge, attitudes, and behaviors, schools must strive to achieve high levels of parent participation and provide parents with multiple opportunities to participate and engage in activities (569).

Provide various formats for involving families and offer frequent opportunities for participation. When a school offers a family activity confined to only one format, the activity is often not successful at attracting high levels of participation (563,564,566,569,570,572,577). Use of multiple formats provides families with options and the ability to choose activities that are interesting and fit their schedule (574,575,588). For example, the purposes of family homework assignments and activity newsletters are to reinforce health and physical education coursework at school, facilitate communication with families about healthy eating and physical activity initiatives at school and within the community, and increase family knowledge of healthy behaviors (e.g., healthy meal preparation and physical family activities) (334,472,479,564,566,567,569–572,574). Although only a few studies have demonstrated that homework activities and newsletters improve student knowledge of and attitudes toward healthy behaviors (566,570) or affect behaviors (569,595), distributing homework and newsletters to families more frequently might increase their effects (569,570).

Family nights are designed to attract families to the school to engage them in health education and promotion activities. This type of event might include skill-building workshops for families on preparing healthy meals or physical activity stations to participate in active games (564,572,574,577). However, participation in family nights is typically low (564,572,577). Internet-based programs might include interactive online activities such as prompts to be physically active or eat a nutritious snack, weight and behavioral assessments, goal-setting, tracking progress toward achieving health goals, and suggestions for overcoming barriers. Internet-based interventions are appealing because parents and children can participate in the program at a convenient time; however, an evaluation of one study found low participation, possibly because of the time required (563).

Two substantial barriers to family participation in school-based programs and activities are scheduling conflicts and lack of transportation. One technique to overcome these barriers is to link health promotion initiatives to activities that already involve family members (580), such as PTA meetings, parent-teacher conferences, tutoring programs, interscholastic sports, and school plays. Schools might consider providing transportation to and offering child care during events (558).

Access Community Resources To Help Provide Healthy Eating and Physical Activity Opportunities for Students

School collaborations with community resources can link students and their families to programs and services that the school is unable to provide independently. Partnerships are beneficial because they conserve resources; reach a wide audience; accomplish objectives of multiple organizations, including schools; increase credibility; improve information sharing; make use of a range of expertise; and foster coordination across sectors of society (*596*). Schools can leverage community resources to offer health promotion activities and events, purchase equipment and safety gear, pay for staff training, create safer environments for play (e.g., safe school yards) and physically active transportation to school (e.g., traffic interventions), attract awareness about healthy lifestyle behaviors, repeat consistent health messages, increase support for school initiatives to promote healthy eating and physical activity, and ensure sustainable funding (*447,583,589,597,598*). Schools also can interact with state and local agriculture through farm-to-school programs. These programs provide local produce, promote and support locally based agriculture, and often connect farmers and students with visits to farms and visits from farmers to the classroom, enabling students to learn how and where food is produced (*599*). Schools also can work with the community to address barriers to healthy eating and physical activity, such as areas that lack access to affordable foods needed for a healthy diet (i.e., food deserts) and a lack of safe places to be active. For example, schools might address food deserts by ensuring that healthy options are offered or available for purchase at all school-sponsored activities (on and off campus) (*600*). Partnerships between schools and local government can create joint-use agreements to use school facilities to host farmers' markets, plant community gardens, or allow public access to school facilities, fitness centers, gymnasiums, or running tracks (*601*).

Involve staff members from universities, hospitals, health centers, and other health organizations in school initiatives on healthy eating and physical activity. Health professionals outside of the school can advise on health education curricula and contribute to lessons and presentations specific to nutrition and physical activity; conduct health screenings; provide expertise on nutrition and physical activity at health fairs, family or teacher workshops, and for health services; and initiate walking and other physical activity initiatives (*592,602*). In 2006, 26% of schools reported working with a local hospital, and 25% reported collaborating with a college or university on school health program activities related to health education (*593*). University faculty members and students

in the health field can provide programmatic and evaluation assistance to schools while gaining practical experience (*603*).

Recruit parent, family, and community volunteers to assist with healthy eating and physical activity initiatives. Parents, other family members, and community members can volunteer their time and skills to support school initiatives and help provide necessary assistance and supervision. For example, families and other community members can supervise school physical activity facilities after regular school hours, allowing for community access to safe and supervised facilities. Volunteers have been shown to be an important component for sustaining programs, even when limited funding is available (*447,584,592*). Schools can offer cost-effective incentives to compensate for volunteers' time (e.g., raffles, door prizes, grocery coupons, T-shirts, childcare, gift cards, discounted trip tickets, transportation tickets, or gas cards) (*604,605*). Parents can relate to volunteers who are also parents, and this networking can be a useful tool for sustaining participation in volunteer programs (*587*). Volunteer groups also can recruit from existing parent networks (such as the PTA) in the school or community.

Link to out-of-school programs that promote healthy eating and physical activity. Out-of-school programs (e.g., after school programs and parks and recreation programs) offer additional opportunities to reinforce health promotion messages taught in schools and can engage students in healthy eating and physical activity (*606*). Such programs can provide health-related experiences that are complementary to the school's curriculum (e.g., opportunities for physical activity, cooking lessons, promoting healthy snacks, farm trips) (*589*). Offering transportation to and from these programs might increase student participation (*574,607*).

Demonstrate Cultural Awareness in Healthy Eating and Physical Activity Practices Throughout the School

Customize activities and communication to reflect the culture of the community. Activities should reflect both the social and environmental aspects of a community (*291,560*). Engaging members from all cultural or language groups represented in the community can foster stronger partnerships among students, families, and community members (*589,594,608*). Policy and program information that is shared with family and community members should be culturally appropriate and translated as needed, with the goal of respecting diverse backgrounds and beliefs (*609*).

Surveying the interests and understanding the culture of families in the community can help schools offer diverse physical activity initiatives that are feasible and aligned with community interests (*588,597,607*). Local markets can provide information about the healthy foods available in the community. Schools should use this information to promote healthy diets and recipes that are feasible for students and their families to incorporate into their lifestyle (*573*). Other factors that can enhance family and community relationships include training of all school staff members in family engagement and hiring staff members and volunteers who reflect the culture of the community (*587*).

Guideline 8. Provide a School Employee Wellness Program that Includes Healthy Eating and Physical Activity Services for All School Staff Members

Nearly 6 million persons work in schools in the United States (*610*). Implementing and sustaining an employee wellness program has the potential to improve staff productivity, decrease employee absenteeism, and decrease employee health-care costs (*611,612*). In addition, employee wellness programs can increase employee morale and improve worker retention and recruitment of new employees (*613,614*). Conversely, employee health risks (e.g., high blood pressure and high cholesterol levels) and lack of participation in worksite fitness and wellness programs are related to higher rates of employee absenteeism (*615*). School employee wellness programs that include healthy eating and physical activity components can increase teacher morale and improve general well-being and perceived ability to handle job stress (*616–618*). A national health objective strives to increase the proportion of worksites that offer an employee health promotion program (objective ECBP 8) (*10*).

Because employee wellness programs might increase healthy eating and physical activity among staff members, these staff members would model positive health behaviors for students (*619,620*). For example, school staff members can have a substantial influence on tobacco-free environments in schools (*621–623*). Students who see teachers smoking during a smoking ban are less likely to adhere to the tobacco-free environment rules (*623*). Furthermore, school staff members are more likely to abstain from use of tobacco on school grounds when they believe that they influence the students' behavior (*621*).

School employee wellness programs typically include health screenings to identify chronic disease risk factors such as high blood pressure or high cholesterol, health education classes, organizational policies that support worksite wellness, and employee assistance programs (*624*). In 2006, 16% of schools offered physical activity and fitness counseling for school staff members, 17% offered nutrition education, and 17% offered weight management services (*624*).

School employee wellness programs for healthy eating and physical activity could include the following components: information and educational activities (e.g., lectures, written materials, and educational software), behavioral strategies (e.g., individual and group behavior counseling, skill-building activities, and rewards or reinforcement), and policy and environmental strategies (e.g., increased access to healthy foods and on-site opportunities for physical activity). *School Employee Wellness: A Guide for Protecting the Assets of our Nation's Schools*, from Directors of Health Promotion and Education, is a step-by-step guide for implementing school employee wellness programs (*625*) (Box 8).

Gather Data and Information To Determine the Nutrition and Physical Activity Needs of School Staff Members and Assess the Availability of Existing School Employee Wellness Activities and Resources

A school employee wellness program should be supported by an environment and a culture that are conducive to health (*618,626–628*). Members of a school employee wellness committee should review organizational policies, programs, strengths, and barriers to identify priorities for nutrition and physical activity (*192,620*).

Determine employee health-related costs. In conjunction with district-level human resources, risk management, and employee benefits staff members, school employee wellness committees can identify critical data related to school employee well-being, such as health insurance costs, workers' compensation claims, absenteeism rates (includes costs of substitute teachers), and employee turnover rates. Analyzing reasons for absenteeism and health insurance claims can assist in identifying health conditions that could be addressed through school employee wellness programs (*625*). Analyzing workers' compensation claims might identify needs for improved worksite safety programs that include physical activity.

BOX 8. Strategies for guideline 8: Provide a school employee wellness program that includes healthy eating and physical activity services for all school staff members

- Gather data and information to determine the nutrition and physical activity needs of school staff members and assess the availability of existing school employee wellness activities and resources.
- Encourage administrative support for and staff involvement in school employee wellness.
- Develop, implement, and evaluate healthy eating and physical activity programs for all school employees.

Assess the status of school employee wellness activities, and identify the nutrition and physical activity interests and needs of school employees. Assessing the current status of school employee wellness activities provides a starting point for planning future programming (*625*). The CDC School Health Index provides a series of items to assess current policies, programs, and practices for school employee wellness. The School Health Index helps schools identify strengths and weaknesses of various components of health promotion for staff members, including health screenings, stress management programs, physical activity and fitness programs, and healthy eating and weight management programs. The School Health Index also includes guidance to develop a plan for improvement (*199,200*). The Community Healthy Living Index (CHILI), developed by the YMCA, is another option for assessing the status of school employee wellness policies and practices (available at www.ymca.net/communityhealthylivingindex/community_healthy_living_index.html). This index contains a series of five assessments that focus on healthy eating and physical activity policies and environmental change strategies in workplaces, schools, and other settings.

Input from school staff members is essential when determining their nutrition and physical activity needs and developing program activities that either influence or affect them personally (*192,628,629*). Using a confidential employee survey is one method for collecting such information. Schools also might consider conducting confidential health screenings for conditions such as high cholesterol or high blood pressure, as well as assessments of employees' eating and physical activity behaviors (*625*). Focus groups and structured interviews also can be used, and direct observations of the school environment can help identify characteristics that influence health-related behaviors (e.g., healthy foods and beverages and bicycle racks) (*630,631*). In addition, schools that establish and sustain school employee wellness programs generally encourage staff members to request activities, classes, and information that are most important for them personally (*619,620,632*).

Encourage Administrative Support for and Staff Involvement in School Employee Wellness

Sharing information with school administrators about the benefits of employee wellness programs and the interests and needs of school staff members can increase their support and resource allocation for such programs (*628,629*).

Obtain administrative support for school employee wellness programs that include healthy eating and physical activity. Administrative support is essential for a school employee wellness program to be viable and sustainable. Administrative support should come from the district superintendent, the principal, and other decision-makers, such as managers or counselors from employee assistance programs, human resource officers, and chief financial officers who oversee annual budgets for school districts. To foster administrator support, schools might consider the following methods (*625*):

- Provide a rationale and demonstrate a need for the program by providing local information and data, such as employee absenteeism rates and reasons for absenteeism.
- Recommend that school administrators attend school wellness conferences offered within their state or by the state education agency.
- Highlight another school or district employee wellness program that has resulted in multiple benefits.
- Develop and deliver a presentation that identifies the need for and benefits of a school employee wellness program in the context of coordinated school health.

Establish a school employee wellness committee, and identify a leader for the committee. An existing committee, such as the school health council or health insurance advisory committee, should have the necessary foundation and components to lead the process of developing a school employee wellness program (*628*). Members of a school employee wellness committee can include (*625*)

- representatives of the people the program will affect, such as bargaining units (e.g., unions), teachers, teacher aides, custodians and maintenance staff members, bus drivers, technology staff members, secretaries, and school nutrition employees;
- representatives from health education, physical education, health services, nutrition services, and mental health and social services;
- an administrator from the school who will communicate with the school board or superintendent or both;
- managers of human resources, employee assistance programs, workers' compensation, benefits, and facilities;
- behavioral change specialists; and
- community representatives from health departments, health care, recreation and fitness centers, businesses, and nonprofit organizations.

The school employee wellness leader can be the school health coordinator or an employee who is committed to offering quality programs for all school staff members. Providing an additional stipend or ensuring that school employee wellness responsibilities are written into a leader's job description might increase the likelihood of sustaining programmatic activities. Such responsibilities can include (*625*)

- coordinating the development, implementation, and evaluation of the program;
- representing school employee wellness on the school health council;

- communicating regularly with administration about the program;
- reporting annually to the school board;
- convening and participating in regularly scheduled meetings of the committee;
- arranging trainings and staff development opportunities;
- communicating with school employees using multiple methods such as e-mail, websites, printed materials, and announcements;
- identifying resources for and scheduling activities;
- developing relationships with community partners; and
- developing and administering the school employee wellness program budget.

Develop, Implement, and Evaluate Healthy Eating and Physical Activity Programs for All School Employees

Establish broad goals and specific objectives for healthy eating and physical activity programs for school employees. A comprehensive school employee wellness program includes goals, objectives, and activities for promoting healthy eating and physical activity. Goals should be realistic and written as broad statements, such as, "increase the proportion of school employees that meet the national physical activity guidelines." Objectives indicate what will be done to achieve the goals; they should be specific, measurable, achievable, relevant, and time sensitive. For example, a physical activity objective might be, "By May 2012, physical activity classes will have been offered once per week for all staff members throughout the entire school year." Various activities to help achieve the objectives and goals should be planned. (e.g., a walking club that meets 1 day per week and is led by a staff member).

Implement activities to promote healthy eating and physical activity that emphasize informational, behavioral skill, and policy and environmental approaches. After a rigorous review of worksite health promotion intervention research, the Task Force on Community Preventive Services recommended worksite obesity prevention and control interventions as an effective method of losing weight. The programs evaluated included at least one of the following components: informational, behavioral, policy, or environmental strategies. Educational activities might include lectures, written materials, and educational software (*378,633*). Behavioral strategies might include individual or group behavioral counseling, skill-building activities, rewards or reinforcement, and inclusion of social support. Policy and environmental strategies should aim to make sustainable organizational changes, such as improving access to healthy foods, providing more on-site opportunities for physical

activities, and point-of-decision prompts that encourage use of stairwells (*378,633*).

Comprehensive environmental, policy, and organizational approaches might result in positive behavior change among school employees. These approaches can include education, employee and peer support for physical activity, physical activity breaks during staff meetings (*634,635*), ongoing incentives for behavior change, access to safe facilities and nutritious foods, and systematic reminders for healthy eating (*636–639*). Use of a pedometer-based physical activity program allows employees to determine their current amount of activity, set goals for improvement, and monitor personal progress (*636,639*).

Evaluate and adapt the school employee wellness program. School employee wellness programs should be evaluated to determine whether objectives have been met, whether employees are satisfied, and what can be done to improve the program. Data and information can be gathered about the process of implementing program strategies and policies. The evaluation also can be used to determine the effects of the program. Questions to consider for assessing the impact include (*625*) the following:

- Have the dietary and physical activity behaviors of employees improved?
- Have health risks such as high cholesterol, overweight or obesity, or high blood pressure decreased?
- Has there been a change in absenteeism?
- Do employees feel that their nutrition and physical activity needs have been met?
- Has there been a noticeable financial effect through reduced health-care costs or other health-related data?

Guideline 9. Employ Qualified Persons, and Provide Professional Development Opportunities for Physical Education, Health Education, Nutrition Services, and Health, Mental Health, and Social Services Staff Members, as well as Staff Members Who Supervise Recess, Cafeteria Time, and Out-Of-School–Time Programs

School staff members who teach physical education or health education, lead nutrition services programs, and implement health, mental health, and social services require certification or specialized training or both (*640–642*). Providing certified and qualified staff members with regular professional development opportunities enables them to improve current skills and acquire new ones (*402,641,643–646*). In addition, staff members who supervise recess, cafeteria time, and out-of-school–time programs can be much more effective if they receive ongoing professional development opportunities. National, state, and local education and health agencies; institutions of higher education; and national and state professional organizations should collaborate to provide professional development opportunities to school health staff members (Box 9).

BOX 9. Strategies for guideline 9: Employ qualified persons and provide professional development opportunities for physical education, health education, nutrition services, and health, mental health, and social services staff members, as well as staff members who supervise recess, cafeteria time, and out-of-school–time programs

- Require the hiring of physical education teachers, health education teachers, and nutrition services staff members who are certified and appropriately prepared to deliver quality instruction, programs, and practices.
- Provide school staff members with annual professional development opportunities to deliver quality physical education, health education, and nutrition services.
- Provide annual professional development opportunities for school health, mental health, and social services staff members and staff members who lead or supervise out-of-school–time programs, recess, and cafeteria time.

Require the Hiring of Physical Education Teachers, Health Education Teachers, and Nutrition Services Staff Members Who Are Certified and Appropriately Prepared To Deliver Quality Instruction, Programs, and Practices

Require the hiring of certified physical education teachers to teach physical education in grades K–12. Schools should develop and adopt policies that require certified physical education teachers, rather than teachers who are certified to teach other subject areas, to teach physical education in grades K–12 to ensure that students receive quality instruction. Certified physical education teachers teach longer lessons, spend more time developing motor and movement skills, impart more knowledge, and provide more moderate and vigorous physical activity than do classroom teachers with little or no specialized training in physical education (*146,383,401,641*). NASPE has established and recommends the National Standards for Beginning Physical Education Teachers, which outlines the areas in which a highly qualified physical education teacher entering the school system should have expertise, including content knowledge,

child and adolescent growth and development, diversity in learning, classroom management and student motivation, communication, planning and instruction, student assessment, reflection, use of technology, and collaboration (*647*). NASPE has produced guidelines for elementary, middle, and high school physical education, which state that physical education should be taught by a qualified teacher with a degree in physical education (for the appropriate grade level) and a current state license to teach physical education (*647–650*).

State and district policies are supportive of hiring qualified physical education teachers. For example, in 2006, all states offered at least one type of certification, licensure, or endorsement to teach physical education (*144*). Many states and districts required newly hired staff members to be certified, licensed, or endorsed by the state to teach physical education. Specifically, 69% of states and 84% of districts had a policy stating that newly hired elementary school physical education teachers be certified, licensed, or endorsed by the state to teach physical education; 88% of states and 87% of districts had such a policy at the middle school level, and 90% of states and 93% of districts had such a policy at the high school level (*144*).

Require the hiring of certified health education teachers to teach health education in grades K–12. Classroom health education teachers who receive specialized training on health education topics have been shown to effectively implement health education programs (*217,651–653*). Certified health education teachers should have the knowledge and skills outlined and recommended in the American Association for Health Education's standards for health education teacher preparation programs. Skills include the ability to assess individual and community health needs; plan, implement, and evaluate health education programs; coordinate health education programs and services; act as a resource person for health education; and communicate health and health education needs, concerns, and resources (*654*).

A national health objective strives to increase the proportion of schools that require newly hired staff members who teach required health education to be certified, licensed, or endorsed by the state in health education (objective EMC 4.2) (*10*). In 2006, 68% of teachers of elementary school classes covering required health instruction and 67% of teachers of required health education courses in middle and high schools were certified, licensed, or endorsed by the state to teach health education at the appropriate grade level (*455*). In 2006, 94% of all states offered some type of certification, licensure, or endorsement to teach health education (*455*). A national health objective also strives to increase the proportion of schools that require newly hired staff members who teach required health education to have undergraduate or graduate training in health education (objective EMC 4.1) (*10*). In 2006, 21% of states and 42%

of districts had a policy stating that newly hired staff members who teach health education at the elementary school level will be certified, licensed, or endorsed by the state to teach health education. In contrast, 72% of states and 70% of districts had this policy at the middle school level, and 79% of states and 83% of districts had this policy at the high school level (455).

Through the certified health education specialist (CHES) program, health education teachers also have the opportunity to gain additional expertise and improve their qualifications. The CHES examination is a competency-based test that measures the possession, application, and interpretation of knowledge related to health education (655). In 2006, 16% of states and 35% of districts had a policy stating that newly hired staff members who teach health education at the middle school level will be CHESs, and 18% of states and 41% of districts had such a policy at the high school level (455).

Require the hiring of qualified nutrition service directors, managers, and staff. Schools should require a minimum level of education and certification for school nutrition professionals to maintain specialized occupational knowledge and expertise. Competencies for school nutrition professionals involve a distinct and complex set of knowledge and skill requirements, such as

- maintaining integrity with federal, state, and local regulations (e.g., use of USDA Foods);
- ensuring that all meals served meet current nutritional standards (e.g., the *Dietary Guidelines for Americans* and meal pattern requirements), including those for children with special needs;
- establishing a leadership role in nutrition education as part of the overall school education program;
- providing a food-safe environment that protects the health and well-being of all school children (e.g., applies principles of the hazard analysis and critical control point system, foodborne illness prevention, and food biosecurity);
- operating effective administrative, procurement, and other financial management protocols to ensure quality food production and distribution;
- implementing a marketing plan for program promotion and creating interest in school meals; and
- managing the school nutrition program staff members according to all federal, state, and local employment regulations, including leadership of professional development opportunities (656,657).

To support such demanding job requirements, school nutrition directors should have, at minimum, a bachelor's degree in a nutrition-related field or food-service management, a dietetics degree, or a certification or credentialing in nutrition services from either the School Nutrition Association or a state program (299). A primary challenge for schools is increasing the

professional qualifications of nutrition services staff members to have the skills needed to provide nutritious and appealing school meals that comply with the *Dietary Guidelines for Americans* and to consistently offer students healthy food and beverage options (658).

State- and district-level education agencies and boards can influence local school practices by establishing professional preparation and certification requirements in addition to offering professional preparation and development opportunities. Nationwide in 2006, 27% of states offered certification, licensure, or endorsement for district nutrition services directors, and 22% of states offered this to school nutrition services managers. Only 16% of all districts required a newly hired school nutrition services manager to be certified, licensed, or endorsed by the state (105). Most districts (57%) required only a high school diploma or its equivalent for newly hired district nutrition services directors; 24% of districts did not have any minimum level of education for newly hired district nutrition services directors; 74% of districts required only a high school diploma or its equivalent for newly hired school nutrition services managers; and 22% of districts did not have any minimum level of education for newly hired school nutrition services staff members. In 2006, only 41% of district-level nutrition services directors and 45% of school-level nutrition services managers reported having an undergraduate degree (105).

Provide School Staff Members with Annual Professional Development Opportunities To Deliver Quality Physical Education, Health Education, and Nutrition Services

Physical education teachers, health education teachers, and nutrition services staff members should receive regular professional development to improve their knowledge, skills, and competencies and be current on the most effective and innovative teaching and programmatic strategies. Quality professional development delivered in group settings, one-on-one, or through communications technology should improve staff knowledge, enable effective implementation of skills and strategies in schools, and positively affect the behaviors of students (659). The National Staff Development Council has developed and recommends the use of standards for professional development that include context standards (e.g., establishment of adult learning communities, improving leadership, and garnering resources), process standards (e.g., using student data to determine staff learning priorities, preparing school staff members to apply research to decision-making, and using learning strategies appropriate to intended goals), and content standards (e.g., preparing school staff members to understand and appreciate all students, create safe environments, and deepen educators' content knowledge and skills) (659).

Comprehensive professional development programs should 1) be based on staff level of knowledge, experience, and needs; 2) model behavior change techniques; 3) provide opportunities to practice; 4) involve multiple sessions so that teachers can practice in classrooms and report on their experiences; and 5) provide opportunities for teachers to share their experiences with peers during posttraining sessions (*640,644,659–662*).

Provide annual professional development opportunities for physical education teachers. Professional development should help physical education teachers provide instruction that meets the interests and skill levels of all students. Physical education teachers should have professional development opportunities that teach concepts of quality physical education instruction, such as how to improve teaching methods, administer fitness tests and assess student performance, encourage family involvement in physical activity, incorporate national or state standards into the curriculum, conduct fitness education, use fitness-oriented technology, and increase active time during physical education class (*145,641,644,663*).

Professional development can enhance teachers' instructional strategies for increasing student physical activity during physical education classes and can enable teachers to develop lesson plans that emphasize student skill development and improve students' enjoyment of being physically active (*383,644,663,664*). Professional development also might influence physical education teachers' personal attitudes and beliefs toward physical activity and fitness (*643,645*).

In 2006, 78% of all states and 91% of all districts provided funding for staff development or offered professional development for physical education teachers on at least one physical education topic (e.g., administering or using fitness tests, student assessment, chronic health conditions, and injury prevention) during the 2 years before the study (*144*). In 2006, physical education teachers from 88% of required physical education classes or courses received professional development on at least one physical education topic. Teachers from at least half of required physical education classes or courses received professional development on injury prevention and first aid, teaching individual or paired activities or sports, teaching movement skills and concepts, and teaching team or group activities or sports. The professional development topics that physical education teachers most reported wanting were teaching methods to promote inclusion and active participation of overweight children, chronic health conditions, using physical activity monitoring devices, helping students develop individualized physical activity plans, and encouraging family involvement in physical activity (*144*). Understanding the differences between what teachers want and what they receive is important to identify any gaps in professional development topics and plan for future trainings or workshops.

NASPE provides various professional development opportunities for physical education teachers. For example, NASPE's Program Improvement in Physical Education (PIPEline) workshop series delivers standards-based training for grades K–12 physical education teachers. Topics covered in PIPEline workshops include instructional practices, assessment strategies, curriculum development, technology integration, and dance instruction in physical education. (Additional information is available at http://www.aahperd.org/naspe.)

Provide annual professional development opportunities for health education teachers. Health education teachers should receive professional development to effectively teach students about foods and nutrients, physical activity, and their connections to health, obesity, and other chronic diseases; to provide students with the knowledge and skills they need to select physical activities they enjoy and healthy foods to prepare; to help students assess their own physical activity and eating habits and plan for change; to identify valid sources of nutrition and physical activity information; to acquire advocacy skills for improving nutrition and physical activity environments; and to facilitate students' ability to identify and correct nutrition and physical activity misconceptions (*462,640,644,660,661,665*).

Professional development also should provide health education teachers with the necessary skills to use innovative, nonlecture techniques, such as active learning strategies, for developing students' knowledge, attitudes, and skills for engaging in healthy eating and physical activity. Strategies that are enjoyable and participatory, emphasize the benefits of healthy eating and physical activity, or provide exposure to new foods and activities are more likely to contribute to student adoption of healthy behaviors (*457,473,666–668*).

Professional development for health education is associated with successful implementation of the classroom curriculum (*217*) and contributes to the implementation of innovative health education methods and techniques (*669*). Health education teachers who receive topic-specific professional development include more instruction on health topics within their lessons than teachers who do not receive topic-specific professional development (*670*).

A national health objective strives to increase the proportion of required health education classes or courses with a teacher who has had professional development related to teaching personal and social skills for behavior change within the past 2 years (objective EMC 4.4) (*10*). In 2006, 88% of states provided funding for or offered professional development on nutrition and dietary behavior, and 82% of states provided funding for or offered professional development on physical activity and fitness during the 2 years before the study. During the same time, 65% of districts provided funding for or offered professional development on nutrition and dietary behavior, an increase from 43% in 2000; and 75% of all districts provided funding for or offered professional development on physical activity and fitness, an increase from 43% in 2000 (455). In addition, approximately half of all districts provided professional development for health education teachers on the following teaching methods: encouraging family or community involvement, teaching skills for behavior change, teaching students with long-term disabilities, using classroom management techniques, and using interactive teaching methods (455). Organizations such as the Rocky Mountain Center's Professional Development Partnership and the Education Development Center (available at http://www.edc.org) provide professional development opportunities that can help schools enhance the delivery of health education curriculum and instruction.

Provide annual professional development opportunities for nutrition services staff members. School nutrition services staff members should receive professional development on topics that support improving the overall school nutrition environment, including healthy food preparation methods; implementing the *Dietary Guidelines for Americans* in school meals (e.g., ensuring that school meals have appealing fruits, vegetables, whole grains, and low-fat or fat-free milk products); competitive food policies; increasing the percentage of students participating in school meals; making school meals more appealing to increase student participation in meal programs; menu planning for healthy meals; preparing fresh fruits and vegetables; food safety; using the cafeteria for nutrition education; offering an array of healthy and culturally appropriate foods and beverages; and reinforcing classroom lessons on healthy food choices in the cafeteria (*105,299,671,672*). Staff training to implement changes within the school meal program can lead to a reduction in calories from total fat, saturated fat, and sodium (*673*). In addition, professional development for nutrition services staff members should also address how to positively influence student food choices at the point of purchase (*642*).

In 2006, two thirds or more of nutrition services managers received professional development on food safety, healthy food preparation methods, personal safety for nutrition services staff members, using hazard analysis and critical control points, selecting and ordering food, and implementing the *Dietary Guidelines for Americans* in school meals during the 2 years before the study. The professional development topics that nutrition service managers reported wanting most were making school meals more appealing, food biosecurity, menu planning for healthy meals, increasing student participation in school meals programs, procedures for food-related emergencies, and using the cafeteria for nutrition education (*105*). Professional

development formats most preferred by nutrition services personnel include hands-on workshops, use of demonstrations, and skill-building workshops with active involvement of participants (*672*).

The USDA Food and Nutrition Service provides strategies for purchasing, preparing, and serving meals aligned with the *Dietary Guidelines for Americans*, including practical tips to update menus and recipes, and suggestions for making changes to help students develop a taste for new menu items (available at http://www.fns.usda.gov/tn/Resources/dgfactsheet_hsm.html). Training opportunities on the provision of healthy school meals are available through the USDA Team Nutrition initiative and the National Food Service Management Institute (available at http://www.fns.usda.gov/tn; http://www.nfsmi.org). The School Nutrition Association also provides its members with professional development training opportunities and certifications in school nutrition (available at http://www.schoolnutrition.org/CareerEducation.aspx).

Provide Annual Professional Development Opportunities for School Health, Mental Health, and Social Services Staff Members and Staff Members Who Lead or Supervise Out-Of-School–Time Programs, Recess, and Cafeteria Time

School health, mental health, and social services staff members and staff members who lead or supervise out-of-school–time programs, recess, and cafeteria time (including staff members from partner organizations such as the YMCA or parks and recreation department) should receive professional development to obtain the skills needed to lead effective programs and educate students on healthy behaviors (*674*). Lack of trained staff is a barrier to implementing safe, organized and effective programs, instruction, and services.

Provide annual professional development opportunities to school health, mental health, and social services staff members. School health, mental health, and social services staff members need preservice and in-service professional development in promoting healthy eating and physical activity and providing healthy eating and physical activity assessment, counseling, and referral. This includes assessing student nutrition, physical activity, and weight status and identifying potential nutrition-related and physical activity-related problems such as eating disorders. Health, mental health, and social services staff members should be equipped with skills to either refer appropriately or assist students with nutrition-related, physical activity–related, or weight-related health problems (*675,676*). In 2006, approximately 43% of school districts provided funding for or offered professional development for health services staff members to provide nutrition and dietary behavior counseling; and 41% of districts provided funding for or offered professional development for physical activity and fitness counseling during the 2 years before the study (*510*). In addition, in 2006, 35% of school districts provided funding for or offered professional development for mental health and social services staff members on nutrition and dietary behavior counseling, and 36% of districts provided funding for or offered professional development on physical activity and fitness counseling during the 2 years before the study (*677*).

For schools implementing BMI measurement programs, health, mental health, and social services staff members must have the appropriate training to obtain accurate and reliable results, ensure privacy and confidentiality, and minimize the potential for stigmatization. Measurements are more likely to be accurate when they are made by trained professionals (*518*).

Provide annual professional development opportunities to staff members who lead or supervise healthy eating and physical activity programs during out-of-school time. Preservice and in-service professional development should help school staff members, coaches, community volunteers, and staff members from partner organizations such as parks and recreation departments plan and implement out-of-school–time healthy eating and physical activity programs that meet a range of student needs and interests. Out-of-school–time programs serving meals or snacks to students need to ensure the provision of nutritious food to give students the energy and nourishment needed to benefit fully from the educational, enrichment, and physical activities being offered. Staff members who work in programs focusing on healthy eating, physical activity, or both in nonschool settings should be adequately trained in providing healthy and nourishing snacks and beverages to participants. Quality professional development should be provided for leaders of out-of-school–time programs to assist them in educating children and adolescents on the importance of making sound decisions about healthy eating and physical activity (*678*).

School staff members, coaches, and community volunteers who lead intramural activities and physical activity clubs during out-of-school time should be trained to place less emphasis on competition and more emphasis on having fun and developing skills. Volunteer coaches who work with beginning athletes in schools should have the level 1 coaching competency delineated by NASPE (*259*) and other professional organizations that provide coaching certification. Like other athletic coaches, volunteer coaches should receive professional development on how to provide experiences for students that emphasize enjoyment, participation, skill development, building confidence, and self-knowledge and also promote healthy behaviors (e.g., healthy eating and adequate fluid replacement). Injury prevention, first aid, cardiopulmonary resuscitation, and precautions

against contamination by bloodborne pathogens are other professional development areas for coaches (*679,680*).

Provide annual professional development opportunities for staff members who lead or supervise recess and cafeteria time. Teachers, school staff members, community volunteers, and staff members from local partner organizations (e.g., local YMCA or parks and recreation departments) who lead or supervise recess should be appropriately trained to provide active supervision, promote physical activity during recess, minimize conflict among students, and maximize cooperation among students. Providing students with various activity choices might maximize physically active time during recess, and working with students to resolve conflict might lead to positive peer interaction during recess and within classrooms.

School staff members supervising cafeteria time should model healthy habits and use appropriate supervisory techniques for managing the school cafeteria. For example, staff members might emphasize good nutrition and healthy eating habits, speak well of the school nutrition program, support social aspects of the meal program (e.g., enjoyment of pleasant conversation, good table manners, and responsible student behavior), and maintain safe, orderly, and pleasant eating environments.

Conclusion

These guidelines were developed through an extensive review of the scientific literature focused on school-based healthy eating and physical activity interventions. Although the scientific interventions highlight what schools can do to address these health behaviors, information is lacking about certain specific intervention strategies that have a long-term effect. For example, the Task Force on Community Preventive Services reported insufficient evidence for school-based nutrition programs and for obesity prevention and control programs in schools. The expert statements and input gathered and reviewed for this report helped contribute to the development of the guidelines and their corresponding strategies. More research could contribute to the strength of these recommendations. Overall, these guidelines provide a comprehensive framework for schools to address healthy eating and physical activity. However, all of these guidelines are not appropriate for every school. Some schools might already be implementing the majority of the guidelines, and other schools might choose to implement only certain guidelines. Prioritizing needs and identifying resources to help implement the guidelines is an important step toward sustaining healthy eating and physical activity policies and practices in schools.

CDC will increase state, territorial, tribal, and local education and health agency awareness of these guidelines through training sessions, conference presentations, webinars, Listservs, and other methods. The findings in this report will help CDC prioritize interventions for school health policies and practices and to identify and develop tools that will assist schools with implementing various components of the guidelines.

Implementing and sustaining school-based healthy eating and physical activity policies and practices will make a substantial contribution toward a healthy future for children and adolescents in the United States. The childhood obesity epidemic and the chronic diseases associated with poor dietary habits and physical inactivity are not likely to be reversed without a strong contribution from schools. Improving and intensifying efforts to promote healthy eating and physical activity is entirely consistent with the fundamental mission of schools: educating young persons to become healthy, productive citizens who can make meaningful contributions to society. School-based policies and practices should be part of coordinated school health programs and reach students from kindergarten through secondary school; prekindergarten programs might also be able to apply these guidelines in their settings. School, district, and state education and health leaders, community leaders, and families can commit to implementing and sustaining healthy eating and physical activity programs within the schools.

References

1. US Department of Health and Human Services. The Surgeon General's call to action to prevent and decrease overweight and obesity. Rockville, MD: US Department of Health and Human Services, Public Health Service, Office of the Surgeon General; 2001.
2. Lichtenstein AH, Appel LJ, Brands M, et al. Diet and lifestyle recommendations revision 2006: a scientific statement from the American Heart Association Nutrition Committee. Circulation 2006;114:84–96.
3. Dietary Guidelines Advisory Committee. Report of the Dietary Guidelines Advisory Committee on the dietary guidelines for Americans, 2010, to the Secretary of Agriculture and the Secretary of Health and Human Services. Washington, DC: US Department of Agriculture, Agricultural Research Service; 2010.
4. Physical Activity Guidelines Advisory Committee. Physical Activity Guidelines Advisory committee report, 2008. Washington, DC: US Department of Health and Human Services; 2008.
5. US Department of Agriculture, US Department of Health and Human Services. Dietary guidelines for Americans, 2010. 7th ed. Washington, DC: US Government Printing Office; 2010.
6. Ogden CL, Carroll MD, Curtin LR, Lamb MM, Flegal KM. Prevalence of high body mass index in U.S. children and adolescents, 2007–2008. JAMA 2010;303:242–9.
7. Daniels S, Arnett D, Eckel R, et al. Overweight in children and adolescents: pathophysiology, consequences, prevention, and treatment. Circulation 2005;111:1999–2012.
8. US Department of Health and Human Services, Public Health Service, Office of the Surgeon General. The Surgeon General's vision for a healthy and fit nation. Washington, DC: US Department of Health and Human Services; 2010.
9. US Department of Health and Human Services. Physical activity guidelines for Americans, 2008. Washington, DC: US Department of Health and Human Services; 2008.
10. US Department of Health and Human Services. Healthy people 2020. Washington, DC: US Department of Health and Human Services; 2010. Available at http://www.healthypeople.gov/2020. Accessed August 18, 2011.
11. CDC. Guidelines for school health programs to promote lifelong healthy eating. MMWR 1996;45(No. RR-9).
12. CDC. Guidelines for school and community programs to promote lifelong physical activity among young people. MMWR 1997;46 (No. RR-6).
13. Green LW. From research to "best practices" in other settings and populations. Am J Health Behav 2001;25:165–78.
14. US Department of Health and Human Services. Physical activity and health: a report of the Surgeon General. Atlanta, GA: CDC; 1996.
15. US Department of Health and Human Services, US Department of Agriculture. Dietary guidelines for Americans, 2005. 6th ed. Washington, DC: US Government Printing Office; 2005.
16. Williams CL, Hayman LL, Daniels SR, et al. Cardiovascular health in childhood: a statement for health professionals from the Committee on Atherosclerosis, Hypertension, and Obesity in the Young (AHOY) of the Council on Cardiovascular Disease in the Young, American Heart Association. Circulation 2002;106:146–60.
17. Kushi LH, Byers T, Doyle C, et al. American Cancer Society guidelines on nutrition and physical activity for cancer prevention: reducing the risk of cancer with healthy food choices and physical activity. CA Cancer J Clin 2006;56:254–81.
18. Xu J, Kochanek KD, Murphy SL, Tejada-Vera B. Deaths: final data for 2007. Natl Vital Stat Rep 2010;58.
19. Mensah GA, Mokdad AH, Ford ES, Greenlund K, Croft J. State of disparities in cardiovascular health in the United States. Circulation 2005;111:1233–41.
20. Thompson PD, Buchner D, Pina IL, et al. Exercise and physical activity in the prevention and treatment of atherosclerotic cardiovascular disease: a statement from the Council on Clinical Cardiology (subcommittee on exercise, rehabilitation, and prevention) and the Council on Nutrition, Physical Activity, and Metabolism (subcommittee on physical activity). Circulation 2003;107:3109–16.
21. Brown L, Rosner B, Willett WW, Sacks FM. Cholesterol-lowering effects of dietary fiber: a meta-analysis. Am J Clin Nutr 1999;69:3042.
22. Ostchega Y, Carroll M, Prineas RJ, McDowell MA, Louis T, Tilert T. Trends of elevated blood pressure among children and adolescents: data from the National Health and Nutrition Examination Survey 1988–2006. Am J Hypertens 2009;22:59–67.
23. Freedman DS, Mei Z, Srinivasan SR, Berenson GS, Dietz WH. Cardiovascular risk factors and excess adiposity among overweight children and adolescents: the Bogalusa Heart Study. J Pediatr 2007;150: 12–7.
24. US Cancer Statistics Working Group. United States cancer statistics: 1999–2007 Incidence and mortality web-based report. Atlanta, GA: CDC, National Cancer Institute; 2010.
25. American Cancer Society. Nutrition and cancer. American Cancer Society; 2007. Available at http://www.cancer.org/downloads/PRO/nutrition.pdf. Accessed June 28, 2011.
26. CDC. National diabetes fact sheet: national estimates and general information on diabetes and prediabetes in the United States, 2011. Atlanta, GA: CDC; 2011.

27. Fox CS, Coady S, Sorlie PD, et al. Trends in cardiovascular complications of diabetes. JAMA 2004;292:2495–9.

28. Hu FB, Stampfer MJ, Solomon CG, et al. The impact of diabetes mellitus on mortality from all causes and coronary heart disease in women: 20 years of follow-up. Arch Intern Med 2001;161:1717–23.

29. US Department of Health and Human Services, National Diabetes Education Program. Overview of diabetes in children and adolescents: a fact sheet from the National Diabetes Education Program. Bethesda, MD: National Diabetes Education Program; 2006. Available at http://ndep.nih.gov/diabetes/pubs/Youth_FactSheet.pdf. Accessed June 28, 2011.

30. SEARCH for Diabetes in Youth Study Group. The burden of diabetes mellitus among US youth: prevalence estimates from the SEARCH for diabetes in youth study. Pediatrics 2006;118:1510–8.

31. American Diabetes Association. Type 2 diabetes in children and adolescents. Pediatrics 2000;105:671–80.

32. Pavkov ME, Hanson RL, Knowler WC, Bennett PH, Krakoff J, Nelson RG. Changing patterns of type 2 diabetes incidence among Pima Indians. Diabetes Care 2007;30:1758–63.

33. Dabelea D, Bell RA, D'Agostino RB Jr, et al. Incidence of diabetes in youth in the United States. JAMA 2007;297:2716–24.

34. Li C, Ford ES, Zhao G, Mokdad AH. Prevalence of pre-diabetes and its association with clustering of cardiometabolic risk factors and hyperinsulinemia among U.S. adolescents: NHANES 2005–2006. Diabetes Care 2009;32:342–7.

35. Institute of Medicine. Preventing childhood obesity: health in the balance. Washington, DC: The National Academies Press; 2004.

36. National Institutes of Health, National Heart, Lung, and Blood Institute. Disease and conditions index: What are overweight and obesity? Bethesda, MD: National Institutes of Health; 2010. Available at http://www.nhlbi.nih.gov/health/dci/Diseases/obe/obe_whatare.html. Accessed June 28, 2011.

37. Krebs NF, Himes JH, Jacobson D, Nicklas TA, Guilday P, Styne D. Assessment of child and adolescent overweight and obesity. Pediatrics 2007;120:S193–228.

38. Barlow SE; Expert Committee. Expert committee recommendations regarding the prevention, assessment, and treatment of child and adolescent overweight and obesity: summary report. Pediatrics 2007;120:S164–192.

39. Hedley AA, Ogden CL, Johnson C, Caroll M, Curtin L, Flegal K. Prevalence of overweight and obesity among U.S. children, adolescents, and adults, 1999–2002. JAMA 2004;291:28407–50

40. Ogden CL, Flegal KM, Carroll MD, Johnson CL. Prevalence and trends in overweight among U.S. children and adolescents, 1999–2000. JAMA 2002;288:1728–32.

41. Ogden CL, Carroll MD, Curtin LR, McDowell MA, Tabak CJ, Flegal KM. Prevalence of overweight and obesity in the United States, 1999–2004. JAMA 2006;295:1549–55.

42. Freedman DS, Kettel Khan L, Serdula MK, Ogden CL, Dietz WH. Racial and ethnic differences in secular trends for childhood BMI, weight, and height. Obes Res 2006;14:301–8.

43. Anderson SE, Whitaker RC. Prevalence of obesity among U.S. preschool children in different racial and ethnic groups. Arch Pediatr Adolesc Med 2009;163:344–8.

44. Miech RA, Kumanyika SK, Stettler N, Link BG, Phelan JC, Chang VW. Trends in the association of poverty with overweight among U.S. adolescents, 1971–2004. JAMA 2006;295:2385–93.

45. Dietz WH. Overweight in childhood and adolescence. N Engl J Med 2004;350:855–7.

46. Guo SS, Chumlea WC. Tracking of body mass index in children in relation to overweight in adulthood. Am J Clin Nutr 1999;70:S145–8.

47. Freedman DS, Kettel L, Serdula MK, Dietz WH, Srinivasan SR, Berenson GS. The relation of childhood BMI to adult adiposity: the Bogalusa Heart Study. Pediatrics 2005;115:22–7.

48. Freedman D, Wang J, Thornton JC, et al. Classification of body fatness by body mass index-for-age categories among children. Arch Pediatr Adolesc Med 2009;163:805–11.

49. Freedman DS, Khan LK, Dietz WH, Srinivasan SA, Berenson GS. Relationship of childhood obesity to coronary heart disease risk factors in adulthood: the Bogalusa Heart Study. Pediatrics 2001;108:712–8.

50. Daniels SR. The consequences of childhood overweight and obesity. Future Child 2006;16:47–67.

51. Olshansky J, Passaro D, Hershow R, et al. A potential decline in life expectancy in the United States in the 21st century. N Engl J Med 2005;352:1138–45.

52. Grundy SM, Cleeman JI, Daniels SR, et al. Diagnosis and management of the metabolic syndrome: an American Heart Association/National Heart, Lung, and Blood Institute scientific statement. Circulation 2005;112:2735–52.

53. Ford ES, Giles WH, Mokdad AH. Increasing prevalence of the metabolic syndrome among U.S. adults. Diabetes Care 2004;27:2444–9.

54. Johnson WD, Kroom JJM, Greenway FL, Bouchard C, Ryan D, Katzmarzyk PT. Prevalence of risk factors for metabolic syndrome in adolescents. Arch Pediatr Adolesc Med 2010;163:371–7.

55. Cook S, Weitzman M, Auinger P, Nguyen M, Dietz WH. Prevalence of a metabolic syndrome phenotype in adolescents: findings from the Third National Health and Nutrition Examination Survey. Arch Pediatr Adolesc Med 2003;157:821–7.

56. US Department of Health and Human Services. Bone health and osteoporosis: A report of the Surgeon General. Washington, DC; 2004.

57. National Osteoporosis Foundation. Boning up on osteoporosis: a guide to prevention and treatment. Washington, DC: National Osteoporosis Foundation; 2003.

58. Taylor G, Theiss P, Mirch MC, et al. Orthopedic complications of overweight in children and adolescents. Pediatrics 2006;1172167–74.

59. Nord M, Andrews M, Carlson S. Household food security in the United States, 2008. ERR-83. Washington, DC: Economic Research Service; United States Department of Agriculture; 2009.

60. Cook J, Frank D. Food security, poverty, and human development in the United States. Ann N Y Acad Sci 2008;1136:193–09.

61. Kaiser LL, Townsend MS. Food insecurity among U.S. children: Implications for nutrition and health. Top Clin Nutr 2005;20:313–20.

62. Alaimo K, Olson CM, Frongillo EA. Food insufficiency and American school-aged children's cognitive, academic and psychosocial developments. Pediatrics 2001;108:44–53.

63. Kleinman RE, Murphy JM, Little M, Pagano J, Wehler CA, Regal K et al. Hunger in children in the United States: potential behavioral and emotional correlates. Pediatrics 1998;101:1–6.

64. Murphy JM, Wehler CA, Pagano M, Little M, Kleinman R, Jellinek MS. Relationship between hunger and psychosocial functioning in low-income American children. J Am Acad Child Adolesc Psychiatry 1998;37:163–70.

65. Murphy JM, Pagano MR, Nachmani J, Sperling P, Kane S, Kleinman RR. The relationship of school breakfast to psychosocial and academic functioning. Arch Pediatr Adolesc Med 1998;152:899–107.

66. Fuller B, Caspary G, Kagan SL, et al. Does maternal employment influence poor children's social development? Early Child Res Q 2002;17:470–97.

67. Casey PH, Szeto KL, Robbins JM, et al. Child health related quality of life and household food security. Arch Pediatr Adolesc Med 2005;195:51–6.

68. Ralston K, Newman C, Clauson A, Guthrie J, Busby J. The National School Lunch Program, background, issues, and trends. ERR-61. Washington, DC: US Department of Agriculture, Economic Research Service; 2008.

69. CDC. Iron deficiency—United States, 1999–2000. MMWR 2002;51:897–9.

70. CDC. Recommendations to prevent and control iron deficiency in the United States. MMWR 1998;47(No. RR-3).

71. US Department of Health and Human Services. Healthy people 2010: with understanding and improving health and objectives for improving health (2nd ed in 2 vols). Washington, DC: US Government Printing Office; 2000.

72. Grantham-McGregor S, Ani C. A review of studies on the effect of iron deficiency on cognitive development in children. J Nutr 2001;131:S64–66.

73. Taras HL. Nutrition and student performance at school. J Sch Health 2005;75:199–213.

74. Cogswell ME, Looker AC, Pfeiffer CM, et al. Assessment of iron deficiency in U.S. preschool children and nonpregnant females of childbearing age: National Health and Nutrition Examination Survey 2003–2006. Am J Clin Nutr 2009;89:1334–42.

75. Nead KG, Halterman JS, Kaczorowski JM, Auinger P, Weitzman M. Overweight children and adolescents: a risk group for iron deficiency. Pediatrics 2004;114:104–8.

76. American Psychiatric Association Task Force on DSM-IV. Diagnostic and statistical manual of mental disorders: DMI-IV. Washington, DC: American Psychiatric Association; 1994.

77. American Psychiatric Association. Practice guideline for the treatment of patients with eating disorders, 3rd ed. Arlington, VA: American Psychiatric Association; 2006.

78. CDC. Youth risk behavior surveillance—United States, 2009. MMWR 2010;59(No. SS-5).

79. Harris EC, Barraclough B. Excess mortality of mental disorder. Br J Psychiatry 1998;173:11–53.

80. US Department of Health and Human Services. Oral health in America: a report of the Surgeon General—executive summary. Washington, DC: US Department of Health and Human Services, National Institute of Dental and Craniofacial Research, National Institutes of Health; 2000.

81. Marshall TA, Levy SM, Broffitt BA, et al. Dental caries and beverage consumption in young children. Pediatrics 2003;112:e184–91.

82. Marshall TA, Eichenberger-Gilmore JM, Broffitt BA, Warren JJ, Levy SM. Dental caries and childhood obesity: roles of diet and socioeconomic status. Community Dent Oral Epidemiol 2007;35:449–58.

83. US Department of Agriculture, Agricultural Research Service. What we eat in America, NHANES 2007–2008. Snacks: distribution of snack occasions. Washington, DC: US Department of Agriculture; 2010. Available at http://www.ars.usda.gov/SP2UserFiles/Place/12355000/pdf/0708/Table_30_DSO_RAC_07.pdf. Accessed June 28, 2011.

84. Briefel RR., Johnson CL. Secular trends in dietary intake in the United States. Ann Rev Nutr 2004;24:401–31.

85. Sacks FM, Svetkey LP, Vollmer VM, et al. Effects of blood pressure on reduced dietary sodium and the Dietary Approaches to Stop Hypertension (DASH) diet. DASH-Sodium Collaborative Research Group. N Engl J Med 2001;344:3–10.

86. Reedy J, Krebs-Smith SM. Dietary sources of energy, solid fats, and added sugars among children and adolescents in the United States. J Am Diet Assoc 2010;110:1477–84.

87. Forshee RA, Anderson PA, Storey ML. Changes in calcium intake and association with beverage consumption and demographics: comparing data from CSFII 1994–1996, 1998 and NHANES 1999–2002. J Am Coll Nutr 2006;25:108–16.

88. CDC. Trends in intake of energy and macronutrients—United States, 1971–2000. MMWR 2004;53:80–2.

89. Enns CW, Mickle SJ, Goldman JD. Trends in food and nutrient intakes by children in the United States. Fam Econ Nutr Rev 2002;14:56–68.

90. Troiano RP, Briefel RR, Carroll MD, Bialostosky K. Energy and fat intakes of children and adolescents in the United States: data from the National Health and Nutrition Examination Surveys. Am J Clin Nutr 2000;72:S1343–53.

91. Enns CW, Mickle SJ, Goldman JD. Trends in food and nutrient intakes by adolescents in the United States. Fam Econ Nutr Rev 2003;15:15–27.

92. Larson NI, Story M, Wall M, Neumark-Sztainer D. Calcium and dairy intakes of adolescents are associated with their home environment, taste preferences, personal health beliefs, and meal patterns. J Am Diet Assoc 2006;106:1816–24.

93. Harnack L, Walter SA, Jacobs DJ. Dietary intake and food sources of whole grains among U.S. children and adolescents: data from the 1994–1996 continuing survey of food intakes by individuals. J Am Diet Assoc 2003;103:1015–9.

94. Neumark-Sztainer D, Wall M, Perry C, Story M. Correlates of fruit and vegetable intake among adolescents. Findings from Project EAT. Prev Med 2003;37:198–208.

95. Zabinski MF, Daly T, Norman GJ, et al. Psychosocial correlates of fruit, vegetable, and dietary fat intake among adolescent boys and girls. J Am Diet Assoc 2006;106:814–21.

96. Larson NI, Neumark-Sztainer D, Hannan P, Story M. Family meals during adolescence are associated with higher diet quality and healthful meal patterns during young adulthood. J Am Diet Assoc 2007;107:1502–10.

97. Van der Horst K, Oenema A, Ferreira I, et al. A systematic review of environmental correlates of obesity-related dietary behaviors in youth. Health Educ Res 2007;22:203–26.

98. Story M, Neumark-Sztainer D, French S. Individual and environmental influences on adolescent eating behaviors. J Am Diet Assoc 2002;102:S40–51.

99. Baker EA, Schootman M, Barnidge E, Kelly C. The role of race and poverty in access to foods that enable individuals to adhere to the dietary guidelines. Prev Chronic Dis 2006;3:A76.

100. Zenk SN, Schulz AJ, Israel BA, James SA, Bao S, Wilson ML. Neighborhood racial composition, neighborhood poverty, and the spatial accessibility of supermarkets in metropolitan Detroit. Am J Public Health 2005;95:660–7.

101. Larson NI, Story M, Nelson MC. Neighborhood environments: disparities in access to healthy foods in the U.S. Am J Prev Med 2009;36:74–81.

102. Powell LM, Slater S, Mirtcheva D, Yanjun B, Chaloupka FJ. Food store availability and neighborhood characteristics in the United States. Prev Med 2007;44:189–95.

103. Bowman SA, Gortmaker SL, Ebbeling CB, Pereira MA, Ludwig DS. Effects of fast-food consumption on energy intake and diet quality among children in a national household survey. Pediatrics 2004;113:112–8.

104. Paeratakul S, Ferdinand DP, Champagne CM, Ryan DH, Bray GA. Fast-food consumption among U.S. adults and children: dietary and nutrient intake profile. J Am Diet Assoc 2003;103:1332–8.

105. O'Toole T, Anderson S, Miller C, Guthrie J. Nutrition services and foods and beverages available at school: results from the school health policies and programs study 2006. J Sch Health 2007;77:500–21.

106. Fox MK, Gordon AR, Nogales R, Wilson A. Availability and consumption of competitive foods in U.S. public schools. J Am Diet Assoc 2009;109:S57–66.

107. Institute of Medicine. Food marketing to children and youth: threat or opportunity? Washington, DC: Institute of Medicine; 2006.

108. Federal Trade Commission. Marketing food to children and adolescents: A review of industry expenditures, activities, and self regulation. Washington, DC, Federal Trade Commission; 2008.

109. CDC. Physical activity levels among children aged 9–13 years—United States, 2002. MMWR 2003;52:785–8.

110. US Department of Transportation Federal Highway Administration. Conference Report on H.R. 3, Safe, Accountable, Flexible, Efficient Transportation Equity Act: A Legacy for Users (SAFETEA-LU). Washington, DC: US Department of Transportation; 2005.

111. Carlson SA, Densmore D, Fulton JE, Yore MM, Kohl HW. Differences in physical activity prevalence and trends from 3 U.S. surveillance systems: NHIS, NHANES, and BRFSS. J Phys Act Health 2009;6:S18–27.

112. Sallis JF, Prochaska JJ, Taylor WC. A review of correlates of physical activity of children and adolescents. Med Sci Sport Exer 2000;32:963–75.

113. Lindquist CH, Reynolds KD, Goran MI. Sociocultural determinants of physical activity among children. Prev Med 1999;29:305–12.

114. Pate RR, Trost SG, Felton GM, Ward DS, Dowda M, Saunders R. Correlates of physical activity behavior in rural youth. Res Q Exerc Sport 1997;68:241–8.

115. Robbins LB, Pis MB, Pender NJ, Kazanis AS. Physical activity self-definition among adolescents. Res Theory Nurs Pract 2004;18:317–30.

116. Walton J, Hoerr S, Heine L, Frost S, Roisen D, Berkimer M. Physical activity and stages of change in fifth and sixth graders. J Sch Health 1999;69:285–9.

117. Sallis JF. Determinants of physical activity behavior in children. In: Pate R, Hohn R, eds. Health and fitness through physical education. Champaign, IL: Human Kinetics; 1994:31–43.

118. Gordon-Larsen P, McMurray RG, Popkin BM. Determinants of adolescent physical activity and inactivity patterns. Pediatrics 2000;105:83-91. Epub June 1, 2000. Available at http://pediatrics.aappublications.org/content/105/6/e83.abstract. Accessed July 1, 2011.

119. CDC. Trends in leisure-time physical inactivity by age, sex, and race/ethnicity—United States, 1994–2004. MMWR 2005;54:991–4.

120. Robbins LB, Pender NJ, Kazanis AS. Barriers to physical activity perceived by adolescent girls. J Midwifery Womens Health 2003;48:206–12.

121. Haverly K, Davison KK. Personal fulfillment motivates adolescents to be physically active. Arch Pediatr Adolesc Med 2005;159:1115–20.

122. Van der Horst K, Paw MJ, Twisk JW, van Mechelen W. A brief review on correlates of physical activity and sedentariness in youth. Med Sci Sport Exer 2007;39:1241–50.

123. Trost SG, Pate RR, Ward DS, Saunders R, Riner W. Correlates of objectively measured physical activity in preadolescent youth. Am J Prev Med 1999;17:120–6.

124. Baker CW, Little TD, Brownell KD. Predicting adolescent eating and activity behaviors: the role of social norms and personal agency. Health Psychol 2003;22:189–98.

125. Frenn M. Determinants of physical activity and low-fat diet among low income African American and Hispanic middle school students. Public Health Nurs 2005;22:89–97.

126. Motl R, Dishman R, Saunders R, Dowda M, Pate R. Perceptions of physical and social environment variables and self-efficacy as correlates of self-reported physical activity among adolescent girls. J Pediatr Psychol 2007;32:6–12.

127. Springer AE, Kelder SH, Hoelscher DM. Social support, physical activity and sedentary behavior among 6th-grade girls: a cross-sectional study. Int J Behav Nutr Phys Act 2006;3:8–18.

128. Voorhees CC, Murray D, Welk G, et al. The role of peer social network factors and physical activity in adolescent girls. Am J Health Behav 2005;29:183–90.

129. Vu MB, Murrie D, Gonzalez V, Jobe JB. Listening to girls and boys talk about girls' physical activity behaviors. Health Educ Behav 2006;33:81–96.

130. Gustafson SL, Rhodes RE. Parental correlates of physical activity in children and early adolescents. Sports Med 2006;36:79–97.

131. Sallis JF, Prochaska JJ, Taylor WC, Hill JO, Geraci JC. Correlates of physical activity in a national sample of girls and boys in grades 4 through 12. Health Psychol 1999;18:410–5.

132. Strauss RS, Rodzilsky D, Burack G, Colin M. Psychosocial correlates of physical activity in healthy children. Arch Pediatr Adolesc Med 2001;155:897–902.

133. Dowda M, Dishman R, Pfeiffer KA, Pate R. Family support for physical activity in girls from 8th to 12th grade in South Carolina. Prev Med 2006;44:153–9.

134. Heitzler CD, Martin SL, Duke J, Huhman M. Correlates of physical activity in a national sample of children aged 9–13 years. Prev Med 2006;42:254–60.

135. Trost S, Sallis J, Pate R, Freedson P, Taylor W, Dowda M. Evaluating a model of parental influence on youth physical activity. Am J Prev Med 2003;25:277–82.

136. Gomez JE, Johnson BA, Selva M, Sallis JF. Violent crime and outdoor physical activity among inner-city youth. Prev Med 2004;39:876–81.

137. Romero AJ, Robinson TN, Kraemer HC, et al. Are perceived neighborhood hazards a barrier to physical activity in children? Arch Pediatr Adolesc Med 2001;155:1143–8.

138. Ferreira I, Van der Horst K, Wendel-Vos W, Kremers S, Van Lenthe FJ, Brug J. Environmental correlates of physical activity in youth—a review and update. Obes Rev 2006;8:129–54.

139. Mota J, Almeida M, Santos R, Ribeiro JC, Santos MP. Association of perceived environmental characteristics and participation in organized and non-organized physical activities in adolescents. Pediatr Exerc Sci 2009;21:233–9.

140. Carver A, Timperio A, Crawford D. Playing it safe: The influence of neighborhood safety on children's physical activity—a review. Health & Place 2008; 14:217-27.

141. Davison KK, Lawson CT. Do attributes of the physical environment influence children's physical activity? A review of the literature. Int J Behav Nutr Phys Act 2006;3:1–17.

142. Cohen L, Davis R, Lee V, Valdovinos E. Addressing the intersection: Preventing violence and promoting healthy eating and active living. Oakland, CA: Prevention Institute; 2010. Available at http://www.preventioninstitute.org/component/jlibrary/article/id-267/127.html. Accessed July 1, 2011.

143. CDC. Barriers to children walking to or from school—United States, 2004. MMWR 2005:949–52.

144. Lee SM, Burgeson CR, Fulton JE, Spain CG. Physical education and physical activity: results from the school health policies and programs study 2006. J Sch Health 2007;77:435–63.

145. McKenzie TL, Sallis JF, Prochaska JJ, Conway TL, Marshall SJ, Rosengard P. Evaluation of a two-year middle-school physical education intervention: M-SPAN. Med Sci Sports Exerc 2004;36:1382–8.

146. Sallis JF, McKenzie TL, Alcaraz JE, Kolody B, Faucette N, Hovell MF. The effects of a 2-year physical education program (SPARK) on physical activity and fitness in elementary school students. Sports, Play, and Active Recreation for Kids. Am J Public Health 1997;87:1328–34.

147. Luepker RV, Perry CL, McKinlay SM, et al. Outcomes of a field trial to improve children's dietary patterns and physical activity. The Child and Adolescent Trial for Cardiovascular Health. JAMA 1996;275:768–76.

148. Nader P, Stone E, Lytle L, et al. Three-year maintenance of improved diet and physical activity: the CATCH cohort. Child and Adolescent Trial for Cardiovascular Health. Arch Pediatr Adolesc Med 1999;153:695–704.

149. Pate R, Ward D, Saunders R, Felton G, Dishman R, Dowda M. Promotion of physical activity among high-school girls: a randomized controlled trial. Am J Public Health 2005;95:1582–7.

150. Andersen RE, Crespo CJ, Bartlett S, Cheskin L, Pratt M. Relationship of physical activity and television watching with body weight and level of fatness among children: results from the Third National Health and Nutrition Examination Survey. JAMA 1998;279:938–42.

151. Coon KA, Tucker KL. Television and children's consumption patterns. A review of the literature. Minerva Pediatr 2002;54:423–36.

152. Crespo C, Smit E, Troiano RP, Bartlett S, Macera C, Andersen R. Television watching, energy intake, and obesity in U.S. children: results from the third National Health and Nutrition Examination Survey, 1988–1994. Arch Pediatr Adolesc Med 2001;155:360–5.

153. Gortmaker SL, Must A, Sobol AM, Peterson K, Colditz GA, Dietz WH. Television viewing as a cause of increasing obesity among children in the United States, 1986–1990. Arch Pediatr Adolesc Med 1996;150:356–62.

154. Hancox RJ, Milne BJ, Poulton R. Association between child and adolescent TV viewing and adult health: a longitudinal birth cohort study. Lancet 2004;364:257–62.

155. Lowry R, Wechsler H, Galuska DA, Fulton JE, Kann L. Television viewing and its associations with overweight, sedentary lifestyle, and insufficient consumption of fruits and vegetables among U.S. high school students: differences by race, ethnicity, and gender. J Sch Health 2002;72:413–21.

156. Utter J, Scragg R, Schaaf D. Associations between television viewing and consumption of commonly advertised foods among New Zealand children and young adolescents. Pub Health Nutr 2006;9:606–12.

157. Viner RM, Cole TJ. Television viewing in early childhood predicts adult body mass index. J Pediatr 2005;147:429–35.

158. Epstein LH, Roemmich JN, Robinson JL, et al. A randomized trial of the effects of reducing television viewing and computer use on body mass index in young children. Arch Pediatr Adolesc Med 2008;162:239–45.

159. Robinson TN. Reducing children's television viewing to prevent obesity: a randomized controlled trial. JAMA 1999;282:1561–7.

160. American Academy of Pediatrics, Committee on Public Education. American Academy of Pediatrics: children, adolescents, and television. Pediatrics 2001;107:423–6.

161. Rideout VJ, Foehr UG, Roberts DF. Generation M: media in the lives of 8- to 18-year-olds. Menlo Park, CA: The Henry J. Kaiser Family Foundation; 2010.

162. Adachi-mejia AM, Longacre MC, Gibson JJ, Beach ML, Titus-Ernstoff LT, Dalton MA. Children with a TV in their bedroom at higher risk for being overweight. Int J Obes 2007;31:644–51.

163. Christakis DA, Ebel BE, Rivara FP, Zimmerman FJ. Television, video, and computer game usage in children under 11 years of age. J Pediatr 2004;145:652–6.

164. Dennison BA, Erb TA, Jenkins PL. Television viewing and television in bedroom associated with overweight risk among low-income preschool children. Pediatrics 2002;109:1028–35.

165. Matheson DM, Killen JD, Wang Y, Varady A, Robinson TN. Children's food consumption during television viewing. Am J Clin Nutr 2004;79:1088–94.

166. Delmas C, Platat C, Schweitzer B, Wagner A, Oujaa M, Simon C. Association between television in bedroom and adiposity throughout adolescence. Obesity Res 2007;15:2495–503.

167. Saelens BM, Sallis JF, Nader PR, Broyles SL, Berry CC, Taras HL. Home environmental influences on children's television watching from early to middle childhood. J Dev Behav Pediatr 2002;23:127–32.

168. Grimm GC, Harnack L, Story M. Factors associated with soft drink consumption in school-aged children. J Am Diet Assoc 2004;104:1244–9.

169. Wiecha JL, Peterson KE, Ludwig DS, Kim J, Sobol A, Gortmaker SL. When children eat what they watch. Arch Pediatr Adolesc Med 2006;160:436–42.

170. American Academy of Pediatrics, Committee on Communications. Children, adolescents, and advertising. Pediatrics 2006;118:2563–9.

171. Coon KA, Goldberg J, Rogers BL, Tucker KL. Relationships between use of television during meals and children's food consumption patterns. Pediatrics 2001;107:E7. Epub January 1. 2001. Available at http://pediatrics.aappublications.org/content/107/1/e7.full. Accessed July 1, 2011.

172. Salmon J, Campbell KJ, Crawford DA. Television viewing habits associated with obesity risk factors: a survey of Melbourne schoolchildren. Med J Aust 2006;184:64-7.

173. Taveras EM, Sandora TJ, Shih M, Ross-Degnan D, Goldmann DA, Gillman MW. The association of television and video viewing with fast food intake by preschool-age children. Obesity Res 2006;14:2034–41.

174. Boynton-Jarrett R, Thomas T, Peterson K, Wiecha J, Sobol A, Gortmaker S. Impact of television viewing patterns on fruit and vegetable consumption among adolescents. Pediatrics 2003;112:1321–6.

175. National Center for Education Statistics. Digest of education statistics: 2004. Washington, DC: National Center for Education Statistics; 2005. Available at http://nces.ed.gov/programs/digest/2004menu_tables.asp. Accessed July 1, 2011.

176. US Department of Education, Institute of Education Sciences. Educational indicators, indicator 24: time in formal instruction. Washington, DC: US Department of Education; 2010. Available at http://nces.ed.gov/pubs/eiip/eiipid24.asp. Accessed July 1, 2011.

177. Dewey JD. Reviewing the relationship between school factors and substance use for elementary, middle, and high school students. J Prim Prev 1999;19:177–225.

178. Dunkle MC, Nash MA. Beyond the health room. Washington, DC: Council of Chief State School Officers, Resource Center on Educational Equity; 1991. Available at http://www.eric.ed.gov/PDFS/ED340681. pdf. Accessed July 1, 2011.

179. Mandell DJ, Hill SL, Carter L, Brandon RN. The impact of substance use and violence/delinquency on academic achievement for groups of middle and high school students in Washington. Seattle, WA: Washington Kids Count, Human Services Policy Center, Evans School of Public Affairs, University of Washington; 2002. Available at http://www.preventionworksinseattle.org/uploads/Impact%20of%20 Substance%20Abuse%20on%20Academic%20Achievement.pdf. Accessed July 1, 2011.

180. Shephard R. Habitual physical activity and academic performance. Nutr Rev 1996;54:S32–36.

181. Kolbe LJ. Education reform and the goals of modern school health programs. The State Education Standard 2002;3:4–11. Epub 2002. Available at http://wvde.state.wv.us/healthyschools/documents/ Education_Reform.pdf. Accessed July 1, 2011.

182. Allensworth D, Lawson E, Nicholson L, Wyche J, eds; Institute of Medicine. Schools and health: our nation's investment. Washington, DC: The National Academies Press; 1997.

183. Kleinman R, Hall S, Green H, et al. Diet, breakfast, and academic performance in children. Ann Nutr Metab 2002;46(Suppl 1): S24–30.

184. Widenhorn-Muller K, Hill K, Klenk J, Wiland U. Influence on having breakfast on cognitive performance and mood in 13- to 20-year old high school students: Results of a crossover trial. Pediatrics 2008;122:279–84.

185. Rampersaud GC, Pereira MA, Girard BL, Adams J, Metzl JD. Breakfast habits, nutritional status, body weight, and academic performance in children and adolescents. J Am Diet Assoc 2005;105:743–60.

186. Hoyland A, Dye L, Lawton CL. A systematic review of the effect of breakfast on the cognitive performance of children and adolescents. Nutr Res Rev 2009;22:220–43.

187. CDC. The association between school-based physical activity, including physical education, and academic performance. Atlanta, GA: US Department of Health and Human Services; 2010. Available at http:// www.cdc.gov/healthyyouth/health_and_academics/pdf/pa-pe_paper. pdf. Accessed July 1, 2011.

188. Marx E, Wooley FS, Northrop D. Health is academic. New York, NY: Teachers College Press; 1998.

189. Fetro JV. Implementing coordinated school health programs in local schools. In: Marx E, Wooley SF, Northrop D, eds. Health is academic. New York, NY: Teachers College Press; 1998:15–42.

190. Cho H, Nadow M. Understanding barriers to implementing quality lunch and nutrition education. J Community Health 2004;29: 421–35.

191. Pateman B, Irvin LH, Shoji L, Serna K. Building school health programs through public health initiatives: the first three years of the Healthy Hawaii Initiative partnership for school health. Prev Chronic Dis 2004;1:A10–6.

192. Valois RF, Hoyle TB. Formative evaluation results from the Mariner Project: a coordinated school health pilot program. J Sch Health 2000;70:95–103.

193. Jones SE, Fisher C, Greene BZ, Hertz MF, Pritzl J. Healthy and safe school environment, part 1: Results from the School Health Policies and Programs Study 2006. J Sch Health 2007;77:522–43.

194. American Cancer Society. Improving school health: a guide to school health councils. Atlanta, GA: American Cancer Society; 1999.

195. Shirer K. Promoting healthy youth, schools, and communities: a guide to community-school health councils. Atlanta, GA: American Cancer Society; 2003.

196. American Cancer Society. Improving school health: a guide to the role of the school health coordinator. Atlanta, GA: American Cancer Society; 1999.

197. Winnail S, Dorman S, Stevenson B. Training leaders for school health programs: the National School Health Coordinator Leadership Institute. J Sch Health 2004;74:79–84.

198. Resnicow K, Allensworth D. Conducting a comprehensive school health program. J Sch Health 1996;66:59–63.

199. CDC. School health index: a self-assessment and planning guide. Middle school/high school version. Atlanta, GA: US Department of Health and Human Services; 2005. Available at http://www.cdc.gov/ HealthyYouth/shi/pdf/MiddleHigh.pdf. Accessed at July 1, 2011.

200. CDC. School health index: a self-assessment and planning guide. Elementary school version. Atlanta, GA: US Department of Health and Human Services; 2005. Available at http://www.cdc.gov/ HealthyYouth/shi/pdf/Elementary.pdf. Accessed July 1, 2011.

201. Austin S, Fung T, Cohen-Bearak A, Wardle K, Cheung LWY. Facilitating change in school health: a qualitative study of schools' experiences using the school health index. Prev Chronic Dis 2006; 3:A35–42.

202. Staten LK, Teufel-Shone NI, Steinfelt VE, et al. The school health index as an impetus for change. Prev Chronic Dis 2006;2:A19–28.

203. Pearlman DN, Dowling E, Bayuk C, Cullinen K, Thatcher AK. From concept to practice: using the school health index to create healthy school environments in Rhode Island elementary schools. Prev Chronic Dis 2005;2 (Spec Issue):A09–A25.

204. Bogden JF. Fit, healthy, and ready to learn: a school health policy guide. Part 1: physical activity, healthy eating, and tobacco-use prevention. Alexandria, VA: National Association of State Boards of Education; 2000.

205. Child Nutrition and WIC Reauthorization Act of 2004, 118 Stat. 729, Sect. 101-502, 108th Cong. (June 30, 2004).

206. Chriqui JF, Schneider L, Chaloupka FJ, Ide K, Pugach O. Local wellness policies: assessing school district strategies for improving children's health 2006–07 and 2007–08. Chicago, IL: Bridging the Gap Program, University of Illinois at Chicago; 2009.

207. Richard B. Russell National School Lunch Act, 42 U.S.C.A. Sect. 1758(b) (2011).

208. US Department of Agriculture. Team nutrition: local wellness policy. Washington, DC: US Department of Agriculture, Food and Nutrition Service; 2004. Available at www.fns.usda.gov/tn/healthy/wellnesspolicy. html. Accessed July 15, 2011.

209. Action for Healthy Kids. Wellness policy development tool. Action for Healthy Kids; 2005. Available at: www.actionforhealthykids.org/ resources_wp.php. Accessed July, 15, 2011.

210. California Project LEAN, The Center for Weight and Health, University of California Berkeley. Policy in action: a guide to implementing your local school wellness policy. Sacramento, CA: California Project LEAN; 2006. Available at http://www.californiaprojectlean.org/doc.asp?id=168. Accessed July 15, 2011.

211. McKenna M.L. Issues in implementing school nutrition policies. Can J Diet Pract Res 2003;64:208-13.

212. CDC. Framework for program evaluation in public health. MMWR 1999;48:1–40.

213. CDC. Physical activity evaluation handbook. Atlanta, GA: CDC; 2002.

214. Muraskin L. Understanding evaluation: the way to better prevention programs. Washington, DC: US Department of Education; 1993.

215. Taras H, Duncan P, Luckenbill D, Robinson J, Wheeler L, Wooley S. Health, mental health, and safety guidelines for schools; 2004. Available at http://www.nationalguidelines.org. Accessed July 15, 2011.

216. Allensworth D. Improving the health of youth through a coordinated school health programme. Promot Educ 1997;4:42–7.

217. Hoelscher D, Feldman H, Johnson C, et al. School-based health education programs can be maintained over time: results from the CATCH institutionalization study. Prev Med 2004;38:594–606.

218. Lytle LA, Ward J, Nader PR, Pedersen S, Williston BJ. Maintenance of a health promotion program in elementary schools: results from the CATCH-ON study key informant interviews. Health Educ Beh 2003;30:503–18.

219. California Department of Education, Advisory Committee on Nutrition Implementation Strategies. School nutrition by design. Sacramento, CA: California Department of Education; 2006.

220. US Department of Agriculture. Guidance for school food authorities: developing a school food safety program based on the process approach to HACCP principles. 4–79. Washington, DC: US Department of Agriculture; 2005.

221. National Food Service Management Institute. Serving it safe. 2nd ed. University, MS: National Food Service Management Institute; 2002.

222. US Department of Agriculture. Changing the scene: improving the school nutrition environment. Alexandria, VA: US Department of Agriculture; 2000.

223. National Coalition for Food Safe Schools. The food-safe schools action guide. Washington, DC: US Department of Health and Human Services; 2005.

224. Conklin MT, Lambert LG, Anderson JB. How long does it take students to eat lunch? A summary of three studies. J Child Nutr Manag 2002; 26:1–6.

225. Bergman EA, Beurgel NS, Englund TF, Femrite A. The relationship of meal and recess schedules to plate waste in elementary schools. J Child Nutr Manag 2004.

226. Tanaka C, Richards KL, Takeuchi LS, Otani M, Maddock J. Modifying the recess before lunch program: a pilot study in Kaneohe elementary school. California J Health Promot 2005;3:1–7.

227. Graham H, Beall DL, Lussier M, McLaughlin P, Zidenberg-Cherr S. Use of school gardens in academic instruction. J Nutr Educ Behav 2005;37:147–51.

228. Morris JL, Zidenberg-Cherr S. Garden-enhanced nutrition curriculum improves fourth-grade school children's knowledge of nutrition and preferences for some vegetables. J Am Diet Assoc 2002;102:91–3.

229. Murphy JM. Education for sustainability: findings from the evaluation study of the edible schoolyard. Berkeley, CA: Center for Eco-literacy; 2003.

230. McAlleese JD, Rankin LL. Garden-based nutrition education affects fruit and vegetable consumption in sixth-grade adolescents. J Am Diet Assoc 2007;107:662–5.

231. Parmer SM, Salisbury-Glennon J, Shannon D, Struempler B. School-gardens: an experiential learning approach for a nutrition education program to increase fruit and vegetable consumption among second-grade students. J Nutr Educ Behav 2009;41:212–7.

232. US Department of Agriculture, Food and Nutrition Service. 2002 Farm Bill, section-by-section summary of provisions affecting child nutrition programs section 4304. Washington, DC: US Department of Agriculture, Food and Nutrition Service; 2008. Available at http://lobby.la.psu.edu/_107th/123_Farm_Bill/Agency_Activities/US_Department_of_Agriculture/USDA_Farm_Bill_Summary_Child_Nutrition_Programs.htm. Accessed July 15, 2011.

233. Richard B. Russell National School Lunch Act, 42 U.S.C.A. Sect. 1758(j) (2011).

234. Harmon A. Farm to school: an introduction for food service professionals, food educators, parents and community leaders. Los Angeles, CA: National Farm to School Program, Center for Food and Justice, Urban and Environmental Policy Institute; 2003. Available at http://www.foodroutes.org/eflyers/FarmtoSchoolGuide.pdf. Accessed July 15, 2011.

235. Robinson-Obrien R, Story M, Heim S. Impact of garden-based youth nutrition intervention programs: a review. J Am Diet Assoc 2009;109: 273–80.

236. Ozer EJ. The effects of school gardens on students and schools: conceptualization and considerations for maximizing healthy development. Health Educ Behav 2007;34:846–63.

237. 42 USCA, 1758(a)(5). 2011.

238. Institute of Medicine. Nutrition standards for foods in schools: leading the way toward healthier youth. Washington DC: Institute of Medicine of the National Academies; 2007.

239. Kaushik A, Mullee MA, Bryant TN, Hill CM. A study of the association between children's access to drinking water in primary schools and their fluid intake: can water be 'cool' in school? Child: Care, Health & Development 2007;33:409–15.

240. Muckelbauer R, Libuda L, Clausen K, Toschke AM, Reinehr T, Kersting M. Promotion and provision of drinking water in schools for overweight prevention: randomized, controlled cluster trial. Pediatrics 2009; 123:e661–3667.

241. Wechsler H, Devereaux RS, Davis M, Collins J. Using the school environment to promote physical activity and healthy eating. Prev Med 2000;31(Suppl):S121–137.

242. Sallis JF, Conway TL, Prochaska JJ, McKenzie TL, Marshall SJ, Brown M. The association of school environments with youth physical activity. Am J Public Health 2001;91:618–20.

243. US Consumer Product Safety Commission. Public playground safety handbook. Washington, DC: US Government Printing Office; 2010. Available at http://www.cpsc.gov/cpscpub/pubs/325.pdf. Accessed July 15, 2011.

244. Olsen HM, Hudson SD, Thompson D. Developing a playground injury prevention plan. J Sch Nurs 2008;24:131–7.

245. Hart JE, Ritson RJ. Liability and safety in physical education and sport. 2nd ed. Reston, VA: National Association for Sport and Physical Education; 2002.

246. National Association for Sport and Physical Education. Guidelines for after-school physical activity and intramural sport programs: a position paper of the National Intramural Sports Council. Reston, VA: National Association for Sport and Physical Education; 2001. Available at http://www.ncpublicschools.org/docs/curriculum/healthfulliving/resources/instructional/intramural-guidelines.pdf. Accessed July 15, 2011.

247. Children's Safety Network at Education Development Center Inc. Injuries in the school environment: a resource guide. 2nd ed. Newton, MA: Education Development Center Inc; 1997.

248. US Department of Education, National Center for Education Statistics, National Forum on Education Statistics; Szuba T, Young R, School Facilities Maintenance Task Force, eds. Planning guide for maintaining school facilities. Washington, DC: National Center for Education Statistics; 2003. Available at http://nces.ed.gov/pubs2003/2003347.pdf. Accessed August 19, 2011.

249. Janda DH, Bir C, Wild B, Olson S, Hensinger RN. Goal post injuries in soccer. A laboratory and field testing analysis of a preventive intervention. Am J Sports Med 1995;23:340–4.

250. Janda DH, Bir C, Kedroske B. A comparison of standard vs. breakaway bases: an analysis of a preventative intervention for softball and baseball foot and ankle injuries. Foot Ankle Int 2001;10:810–6.

251. Janda DH. The prevention of baseball and softball injuries. Clin Orthop Relat Res 2003;409:20–8.

252. Heck JF, Clarke KS, Peterson TR, Torg JS, Weis MP. National Athletic Trainers' Association position statement: head-down contact and spearing in tackle football. J Athl Train 2004;39:101–11.

253. Jones NP. Eye injury in sport. Sports Med 1989;7:163–81.

254. Jambor T, Palmer SD. Playground safety manual. Birmingham, AL: Alabama Chapter of the American Academy of Pediatrics; 1991.

255. CDC. Promising practice in chronic disease prevention: a public health framework for action. Atlanta, GA: US Department of Health and Human Services; 2003.

256. Veigel JD, Pleacher MD. Injury prevention in youth sports. Curr Sports Med Rep 2008;7:348–52.

257. McKeag DB, Moeller JL. Preparticipation screening. In: McKeag DB, Moeller JL, eds. ACSM's primary care sports medicine. 2nd ed. Philadelphia, PA: Lippincott Williams & Wilkins; 2007:55–80.

258. Demorest RA, Landry GL. Training issues in elite young athletes. Curr Sports Med Rep 2004;3:167–72.

259. National Association for Sport and Physical Education. National standards for athletic coaches. Reston, VA: National Association for Sport and Physical Education; 2006.

260. National Association for Sport and Physical Education. Eight domains of coaching competencies. Reston, VA: National Association for Sport and Physical Education; 2006.

261. Saluja G, Marshall SW, Gilchrist J, Schroeder T. Sports and recreational injuries. In: Liller K, ed. Injury prevention for children and adolescents: integration of research, practice, and advocacy. 1st ed. Washington, DC: American Public Health Association; 2006:233–60.

262. Schwebe DC. Safety on the playground: mechanisms through which adult supervision might prevent playground injury. J Clin Psychol Med S 2006;13:135–43.

263. National Program for Playground Safety. S.A.F.E. playground supervision kit. Cedar Falls, IA: National Program for Playground Safety; 2002.

264. Evenson KR, McGinn AP. Availability of school physical activity facilities to the public in four U.S. communities. Am J Health Promot 2004;18:243–50.

265. Farley TA, Meriweather RA, Baker ET, Watkins LT, Johnson CC, Webber LS. Safe places to promote physical activity in inner-city children: results from a pilot study of an environmental intervention. Am J Public Health 2007;97:1625–31.

266. Spengler JO, Young SJ, Linton LS. Schools as a community resource for physical activity: legal considerations for decision makers. Am J Health Promot 2007;21:390–6.

267. Choy LB, McGurk MD, Tamashiro R, Nett B, Maddock JE. Increasing access to places for physical activity through a joint use agreement: a case study in urban Honolulu. Prev Chronic Dis 2008;5.

268. Food and Nutrition Service, US Department of Agriculture; CDC, US Department of Health and Human Services; US Department of Education. Making it happen: school nutrition success stories. Alexandria, VA: US Department of Agriculture; 2005.

269. French SA. Pricing effects on food choices. J Nutr 2003;133:S841–3.

270. Shannon C, Story M, Fulkerson JA, French SA. Factors in the school cafeteria influencing food choices by high school students. J Sch Health 2002;72:229–34.

271. French SA, Wechsler H. School-based research and initiatives: fruit and vegetable environment, policy, and pricing workshop. Prev Med 2004;39(Suppl 2):S101–107.

272. French SA, Story M, Jeffery RW, et al. Pricing strategy to promote fruit and vegetable purchase in high school cafeterias. J Am Diet Assoc 1997;97:1008–10.

273. French SA, Jeffery RW, Story M, et al. Pricing and promotion effects on low-fat vending snack purchases: the CHIPS study. Am J Public Health 2001;91:112–7.

274. Hannan P, French SA, Story M, Fulkerson JA. A pricing strategy to promote sales of lower fat foods in high school cafeterias: acceptability and sensitivity analysis. Am J Health Promot 2002;17:1–6.

275. Baxter SD. Are elementary schools teaching our children to prefer candy but not vegetables? J Sch Health 1998;68:111–3.

276. Birch LL. Development of food preferences. Annu Rev Nutr 1999;19:41–62.

277. Fisher J, Birch L. Restricting access to palatable foods affects children's behavioral response, food selection, and intake. Am J Clin Nutr 1999;69:1264–72.

278. Puhl RM, Schwartz MB. If you are good you can have a cookie: How memories of childhood food rules link to adult eating behaviors. Eat Behav 2003;4:283–93.

279. National Association for Sport and Physical Education. What constitutes a quality physical education program? Reston, VA: National Association for Sport and Physical Education; 2003.

280. Jarrett OS, Maxwell DM, Dickerson C, Hoge P, Davies G, Yetley A. Impact of recess on classroom behavior: group effects and individual differences. J Educ Res 1998;92:121–6.

281. Pellegrini AD, Davis PD. Relations between children's playground and classroom behaviour. Br J Educ Psychol 1993;63:89–95.

282. Eisenberg ME, Neumark-Sztainer D, Story M. Associations of weight-based teasing and emotional well-being among adolescents. Arch Pediatr Adolesc Med 2003;157:733–8.

283. Michigan Department of Education. The role of Michigan schools in promoting healthy weight: a consensus paper. Lansing, MI: Michigan Department of Education; 2001. Available at http://www.michigan.gov/documents/healthyweight_13649_7.pdf. Accessed July 15, 2011.

284. National Association for Sport and Physical Education. Position on dodgeball in physical education. Reston, VA: National Association for Sport and Physical Education; 2004.

285. Discrimination Prohibited, 7 C.F.R. Sect. 15.3 (2011).

286. US Department of Agriculture, Food and Nutrition Service. Accommodating children with special dietary needs in the school nutrition programs: guidance for school food service staff. Alexandria, VA: US Department of Agriculture; 2001.

287. Wilson TK, Bogden JF. Fit, healthy, and ready to learn, part III: policies related to asthma, school health services, and healthy environments. Alexandria, VA: National Association of State Boards of Education; 2005.

288. Block ME, Garcia C. Including students with disabilities in regular physical education. Block ME, Garcia C, eds. Reston, VA: National Association for Sport and Physical Education, American Association for Active Lifestyle and Fitness; 1995

289. American Dietetic Association. Position of the American Dietetic Association: individual-, family-, school-, and community-based interventions for pediatric overweight. J Am Diet Assoc 2006; 106:925–45.

290. Durstine JL, Pinter P, Franklin BA, Morgan D, Pitetti KH, Roberts SO. Physical activity for the chronically ill and disabled. Sports Med 2000;30:207–19.

291. Flynn MA, McNeil DA, Maloff B, et al. Reducing obesity and related chronic disease risk in children and youth: a synthesis of evidence with 'best practice' recommendations. Obes Rev 2006;7:7–66.

292. Fulton JE, Garg M, Galuska DA, Rattay KT, Caspersen CJ. Public health and clinical recommendations for physical activity and physical fitness: Special focus on overweight youth. Sports Med 2004;34: 581–99.

293. National Association for Sport and Physical Education. Moving into the future: national standards for physical education. 2nd ed. Reston, VA: National Association for Sport and Physical Education; 2004.

294. National Asthma Education and Prevention Program. Students with chronic illnesses: guidance for families, schools, and students. J Sch Health 2003;73:131–2.

295. Oude Luttikhuis H, Baur L, Jansen H, et al. Interventions for treating obesity in children. CD001872. Cochrane Database Systematic Review; 2003.

296. National Asthma Education and Prevention Program. Breathing difficulties related to physical activity for students with asthma: exercise-induced asthma. Bethesda, MD: National Asthma Education and Prevention Program; National Heart, Lung, and Blood Institute; 2005.

297. National Heart Lung and Blood Institute. Expert panel report 3: guidelines for the diagnosis and management of asthma. 08-4051. Bethesda, MD: National Institutes of Health, US Department of Health and Human Services; 2007.

298. American Dietetic Association. Position of the American Dietetic Association: local support for nutrition integrity in schools. J Am Diet Assoc 2006;106:122–3.

299. American Dietetic Association; Society for Nutrition Education; American School Food Service Association. Position of the American Dietetic Association, Society for Nutrition Education, and American School Food Service Association. Nutrition services: an essential component of comprehensive school health programs. J Nutr Educ Behav 2003;35:57–67.

300. Birch LL, Fisher JO. Development of eating behaviors among children and adolescents. Pediatrics 1998;101:539–49.

301. Perry CL, Bishop DB, Taylor GL, et al. A randomized school trial of environmental strategies to encourage fruit and vegetable consumption among children. Health Educ Behav 2004;31:65–76.

302. Gordon AR, Cohen R, Crepinsek MK, Fox MK, Hall J, Zeidman E. The Third School Nutrition Dietary Assessment Study: background and study design. J Am Diet Assoc 2009;109(Suppl 2):S20–30.

303. United States Department of Agriculture. National School Lunch Program: participation and lunches served. Washington, DC: US Department of Agriculture; 2011. Available at http://www.fns.usda.gov/pd/slsummar.htm. Accessed July 15, 2011.

304. US Department of Agriculture. School breakfast program participation and meals served. United States Department of Agriculture; 2011. Available at http://www.fns.usda.gov/pd/sbsummar.htm. Accessed July 15, 2011.

305. Briefel RR, Wilson A, Gleason P. Consumption of low-nutrient, energy-dense foods and beverages at school, home, and other locations among school lunch participants and nonparticipants. J Am Diet Assoc 2009;109(Suppl 2):S79–90.

306. Condon EM, Crepinsek MK, Fox MK. School meals: types of foods offered to and consumed by children at lunch and breakfast. J Am Diet Assoc 2009;109(Suppl 2):S67–78.

307. Gordon AR, Crepinsek MK, Briefel RR, Clark MA, Fox MK. The third school nutrition dietary assessment study: summary and implications. J Am Diet Assoc 2009;109(Suppl 1):S129–135.

308. Clark MA, Fox MK. Nutritional quality of the diets of U.S. public school children and the role of the school meals program. J Am Diet Assoc 2009;109(Suppl 2):S44–56.

309. Gleason PM, Dodd AH. School breakfast program but not school lunch program participation is associated with lower body mass index. J Am Diet Assoc 2009;109(Suppl 2):S118–28.

310. Murphy JM, Pagano M, bishop SJ. Impact of a universally-free, in-classroom school breakfast program on achievement: results from the Abell Foundation's Baltimore Breakfast Challenge Program. Boston, MA: Massachusetts General Hospital; 2001.

311. Murphy JM, Drake JE, Weineke KM. Academics and breakfast connection pilot: final report on New York's Classroom Breakfast Project. Albany, NY: Nutrition Consortium of New York; 2005.

312. Powell CA, Walker SP, Chang SM, Grantham-McGregor SM. Nutrition and education: a randomized trial of the effects of breakfast in rural primary school children. Am J Clin Nutr 1998;68:873–9.

313. Meyers A, Sampson A, Weitzman M, Rogers B, Kayne H. School breakfast program and school performance. Am J Dis Child 1989; 143:1234–9.

314. US Department of Agriculture, Food and Nutrition Service; Gordon A, Fox MK, Clark M, et al, eds. School Nutrition Dietary Assessment Study—III, vol II: student participation and dietary intakes. CN-07-SNDA-III. Alexandria, VA: US Department of Agriculture; 2007.

315. Bernstein LS, McLaughlin JE, Crepins MK, Daft IM. Evaluation of the school breakfast program pilot project: final report. Alexandria, VA: US Department of Agriculture; 2004.

316. Determining Eligibility for Free and Reduced Price Meals and Free Milk in Schools, 7 C.F.R. Sect. 245 (2011).

317. Kennedy E, Davis C. U.S. Department of Agriculture school breakfast program. Am J Clin Nutr 1998;67(Suppl):S798–803.

318. Healthy, Hunger-Free Kids Act of 2010. PL 111-296, 201. 12-13-2010. 124 Stat 3183.

319. Institute of Medicine. School meals: building blocks for healthy children. Washington, DC: The National Academies Press; 2010.

320. Richard B. Russell National School Lunch Act, 42 U.S.C.A. Sect. 1758(h) (2011).

321. Crepinsek MK, Gordon AR, McKinney PM, Condon EM, Wilson A. Meals offered and served in U.S. public schools: do they meet nutrient standards? J Am Diet Assoc 2009;109(Suppl 1):S31–43.

322. US Department of Agriculture, Food and Nutrition Service. A menu planner for healthy school meals. Washington, DC: US Department of Agriculture; 1998

323. US Government Accountability Office. School meal programs: revenue and expense information from selected states. GAO-03-569. Washington, DC: US Government Accountability Office; 2003.

324. Mississippi Department of Education, Office of Healthy School and Child Nutrition Programs. Nutrition integrity in Mississippi schools, replacing kitchen fryers with combination oven steamers: six steps to success. Mississippi Department of Education, Office of Healthy Schools and Child Nutrition Programs; 2008.

325. Roberts SM, Pobocik RS, Deek R, Besfrove A, Prostine BA. A qualitative study of junior high school principals' and school food service directors' experiences with the Texas school nutrition policy. J Nutr Educ Behav 2009;41:293–9.

326. Brown DM. Prevalence of food production systems in school foodservice. J Am Diet Assoc 2005;105:1261–5.

327. Lambert LG, Raidl M, Carr DH, Safaii S, Tidwell DK. School nutrition directors' and teachers' perceptions of the advantages, disadvantages, and barriers to participation in the school breakfast program. J Child Nutr Manag 2007;31.

328. Sallis JF, McKenzie TL, Conway TL, et al. Environmental interventions for eating and physical activity: a randomized controlled trial in middle schools. Am J Prev Med 2003;24:209–17.

329. US Department of Agriculture. School lunch and breakfast cost study—II, final report. Washington, DC: US Department of Agriculture; 2008.

330. Wagner B, Senauer B, Runge CF. An empirical analysis of and policy recommendations to improve the nutritional quality of school meals. Rev Agric Econ 2007;29:672–88.

331. Almanza B. Equipment purchasing and facility design for school nutrition programs. R-131-08 (GY05). University, MS: University of Mississippi, National Food Service Management Institute; 2009.

332. US Department of Agriculture. The road to SMI success—a guide for school foodservice directors. Washington, DC: US Department of Agriculture; 2007.

333. O'Neil CE, Nicklas TA. Gimme 5: an innovative, school-based nutrition intervention for high school students. J Am Diet Assoc 2002;102(Suppl 3):S93–6.

334. Story M, Mays Warren R, Bishop D, et al. 5-a-day power plus: process evaluation of a multicomponent elementary school program to increase fruit and vegetable consumption. Health Educ Behav 2000;27:187–200.

335. Zive MM, Pelletier RL, Sallis JF, Elder JP. An environmental intervention to improve a la carte foods at middle schools. J Am Diet Assoc 2002;102(Suppl 3):S76–8.

336. National Food Service Management Institute. Culinary techniques for healthy school meals. 2nd ed. University, MS: National Food Service Management Institute; 2009.

337. Gorski-Berry DM. Wrapping it all up: the value of packaging. J Dairy Sci 1999;82:2257–8.

338. National School Lunch Program, Competitive Food Services, 7 C.F.R. Sect. 210.11 (2011).

339. School Breakfast Program, Competitive Food Services, 7 C.F.R. Sect. 220.12 (2011).

340. National School Lunch Program, Categories of Foods of Minimal Nutritional Value, 7 C.F.R. Sect. 210 App. B (2011).

341. School Breakfast Program, Categories of Foods of Minimal Nutritional Value, 7 C.F.R. Sect. 220 App. B (2011).

342. Child Nutrition Act of 1966, 42 U.S.C.A. Sect. 1779(b) (2011).

343. CDC. Competitive foods and beverages in U.S. schools—a state policy analysis, October 2010. Atlanta, GA, CDC; In press 2011.

344. US Government Accountability Office. School meal programs: competitive foods are widely available and generate substantial revenues for schools. GAO-050563. Washington, DC: US Government Accountability Office; 2005.

345. Abraham SM, Chattopadhvav M, Montgomery M, Steiger DM, Daft B. The School Meals Initiative Implementation Study—third year report. Nutrition Assistance Program Report Series CN02-SMI3. Alexandria, VA: US Department of Agriculture, Food and Nutrition Service, Office of Analysis, Nutrition and Evaluation; 2002.

346. CDC. Competitive foods and beverages available for purchase in secondary schools—selected sites, United States, 2006. MMWR 2008;57:935–38.

347. Brener ND, McManus T, Foti K, et al. School health profiles 2008: characteristics of health programs among secondary schools. Atlanta, GA: CDC; 2009.

348. Fox MK, Dodd AH, Wilson A, Gleason PM. Association between school food environment and practices and body mass index of U.S. public school children. J Am Diet Assoc 2009;109(Suppl 2):S108–17.

349. Briefel RR, Crepinsek MK, Cabili C, Wilson A, Gleason PM. School food environments and practices affect dietary behaviors of U.S. public school children. J Am Diet Assoc 2009;109(Suppl 2):S91–107.

350. Gonzalez W, Jones SJ, Frongillo EA. Restricting snacks in U.S. elementary schools is associated with higher frequency of fruit and vegetable consumption. J Nutr 2009;139:142–4.

351. US Department of Agriculture. Foods sold in competition with USDA meal programs: a report to Congress. Washington, DC: US Department of Agriculture; 2001.

352. Kubik M, Lytle L, Hannan P, Perry C, Story M. The association of the school food environment with dietary behaviors of young adolescents. Am J Public Health 2003;93:1168–73.

353. Kubik M, Lytle L, Story M. Schoolwide food practices are associated with body mass index in middle school students. Arch Pediatr Adolesc Med 2005;159:1111–4.

354. US Department of Agriculture, Food and Nutrition Service; Fox MK, Crepinsek MK, Connor P, Battaglia M, eds. School nutrition dietary assessment study—II: summary of findings. Alexandria, VA: US Department of Agriculture; 2001.

355. French SA, Story M, Fulkerson JA, Hannan P. An environmental intervention to promote lower-fat food choices in secondary schools: outcomes of the TACOS Study. Am J Public Health 2004;94:1507–12.

356. Jones SJ, Gonzalez W, Frongillo EA. Policies that restrict sweetened beverage availability may reduce consumption in elementary-school children. Pub Health Nutr 2009;13:589–95.

357. Snelling AM, Kennard T. The impact of nutrition standards on competitive food offerings and purchasing behaviors of high school students. J Sch Health 2009;79:541–6.

358. Richard B. Russell National School Lunch Act, 42 U.S.C.A. Sect. 1758(b)(2) (2011).

359. Wharton CM, Long M, Schwartz MB. Changing nutrition standards in schools: the emerging impact on school revenue. J Sch Health 2008;78:245–51.

360. Wojcicki J, Heyman MB. Healthier choices and increased participation in a middle school lunch program: effects of nutrition policy changes in San Francisco. Am J Public Health 2006;96:1542–7.

361. Center for Weight and Health, University of California, Berkeley. Pilot implementation of SB 19 in California middle and high schools: report on accomplishments, impact, and lessons learned. Berkeley, CA: University of California, Berkeley; 2005.

362. West Virginia University, Robert C. Byrd Health Sciences Center, Health Research Center. West Virginia Healthy Lifestyles Act: year one evaluation report. Morgantown, WV: West Virginia University; 2009.

363. Connecticut State Department of Education. Summary data report on Connecticut's healthy snack pilot. Hartford, CT: Connecticut State Department of Education; 2006.

364. Brown DM, Tammineni SK. Managing sales of beverages in schools to preserve profits and improve children's nutrition intake in 15 Mississippi schools. J Am Diet Assoc 2009;109:2036–42.

365. Johnston LD, Delvaux K, O'Malley PM. Soft drink availability, contracts, and revenues in American secondary schools. Am J Prev Med 2007;33(Suppl 4):S209–225.

366. Greves MH, Rivara F. Report card on school snack food policies among the United States' largest school districts in 2004–2005: room for improvement. Int J Behav Nutr Phys Act 2006;3:1.

367. Fulkerson JA, French SA, Story M, Nelson H, Hannan PJ. Promotions to increase lower-fat food choices among students in secondary schools: description of outcomes of TACOS (Trying Alternative Cafeteria Options in Schools). Public Health Nutr 2004;7:665–74.

368. Cullen KW, Thompson VJ, Watson K, Nicklas T. Marketing fruits and vegetables to middle school students: formative assessment results. J Child Nutr Manag 2005;29.

369. Davis EM, Cullen KW, Watson KB, Konarik M, Radcliffe J. A fresh fruit and vegetable program improves high school students' consumption of fresh produce. J Am Diet Assoc 2009;109:1227–31.

370. Food and Nutrition Service. Fruits and vegetables galore: helping kids eat more. Washington, DC: US Department of Agriculture; 2004.

371. Just DR, Mancino L, Wansink B. Could behavioral economics help improve diet quality for nutrition assistance program participants? Washington, DC: US Department of Agriculture; 2007.

372. US Department of Agriculture, Food and Nutrition Service. Fruit and vegetable program handbook. Washington, DC: US Department of Agriculture; 2008.

373. The Food Trust. Food Trust healthy food toolkit. Philadelphia, PA: The Food Trust; Available at http://www.thefoodtrust.org/php/programs/comp.school.nutrition.php. Accessed July 15, 2011.

374. Nemours Health and Prevention Services. Planting the seeds for healthy schools: building effective district wellness policies. Jacksonville, FL: Nemours Health and Prevention Services; 2008.

375. Kubik M, Lytle L, Farbakhsh K, Moe S, Samuelson A. Food use in middle and high school fundraising: Does policy support healthful practice? Results from a survey of Minnesota school principals. J Am Diet Assoc 2009;109:1215–19.

376. National Association for Sport and Physical Education. Is it physical education or physical activity?: understanding the difference. Reston, VA: National Association for Sport and Physical Education; 2005. Available at http://www.aahperd.org/naspe/publications/teachingTools/PAvsPE.cfm. Accessed July 15, 2011.

377. National Association for Sport and Physical Education. Comprehensive school physical activity programs. Reston, VA: National Association for Sport and Physical Education; 2008. Available at http://www.aahperd.org/naspe/standards/upload/Comprehensive-School-Physical-Activity-Programs-2008.pdf. Accessed July 15, 2011.

378. Kahn EB, Ramsey LT, Brownson RC, et al. The effectiveness of interventions to increase physical activity. A systematic review. Am J Prev Med 2002;22(Suppl 4):S73–107.

379. National Association for Sport and Physical Education. Physical education is critical to a complete education. Reston, VA: National Association for Sport and Physical Education; 2001. Available at http://www.aahperd.org/naspe/standards/upload/Physical-Education-is-Critical-to-a-Complete-Education-2001.pdf. Accessed July 15, 2011.

380. Trudeau F, Shephard RJ. Contribution of school programmes to physical activity levels and attitudes in children and adults. Sports Med 2005;35:89–105.

381. Donnelly JE, Jacobsen DJ, Whatley JE, et al. Nutrition and physical activity program to attenuate obesity and promote physical and metabolic fitness in elementary school children. Obes Res 1996;4:229–43.

382. McKenzie TL, Nader PR, Strikmiller PK, et al. School physical education: effect of the Child and Adolescent Trial for Cardiovascular Health. Prev Med 1996;25:423–31.

383. McKenzie TL, Marshall SJ, Sallis JF, Conway TL. Student activity levels, lesson context, and teacher behavior during middle school physical education. Res Q Exerc Sport 2000;71:249–59.

384. Dishman RK, Motl RW, Saunders R, et al. Enjoyment mediates effects of a school-based physical-activity intervention. Med Sci Sports Exerc 2005;37:478–87.

385. National Association for Sport and Physical Education. Opposing substitution and waiver/exemptions for required physical education. Reston, VA: National Association for Sport and Physical Education; 2006. Available at http://www.aahperd.org/naspe/standards/upload/Opposing-Substition-Waiver-Exemptions-for-Required-PE-2006.pdf. Accessed July 15, 2011.

386. Ayers SF. High school students' physical education conceptual knowledge. Res Q Exerc Sport 2004;75:272–87.

387. Dale D, Corbin CB. Physical activity participation of high school graduates following exposure to conceptual or traditional physical education. Res Q Exerc Sport 2000;71:61–8.

388. Fardy PS, White RE, Haltiwanger-Schmitz K, et al. Coronary disease risk factor reduction and behavior modification in minority adolescents: the PATH program. J Adolesc Health 1996;18:247–53.

389. CDC. Physical education curriculum analysis tool. Atlanta, GA: US Department of Health and Human Services; 2006. Available at http://www.cdc.gov/healthyyouth/pecat/pdf/PECAT.pdf. Accessed July 15, 2011.

390. Pellett TL, Blakemore CL. Comparisons of teaching presentation and development of content: implications for effectiveness of teaching. Percept Mot Skills 1997;85:963–72.

391. Karabourniotis D, Evaggelinou C, Tzetzis G, Kourtessis T. Curriculum enrichment with self-testing activities in development of fundamental movement skills of first-grade children in Greece. Percept Mot Skills 2002;94:1259–70.

392. Ernst M, Beighle A, Corbin CB, Pangrazi R. Appropriate and inappropriate uses of Fitnessgram: A commentary. J Phys Act Health 2006;3(Suppl 2):S90–100.

393. Twisk JW, Kemper HC, van Mechelen W. The relationship between physical fitness and physical activity during adolescence and cardiovascular disease risk factors at adult age. The Amsterdam Growth and Health Longitudinal Study (AGAHLS). Int J Sports Med 2002;23(Suppl 1):S8–14.

394. Pangrazi R. Dynamic physical education for elementary school students. 15th ed. London, England: Benjamin Cummings; 2006.

395. Whitehead JR, Eklund RC, Williams AC. Using skinfold calipers while teaching body fatness-related concepts: cognitive and affective outcomes. J Sci Med Sport 2003;6:461–76.

396. Bouchard C, Daw EW, Rice T, et al. Familial resemblance for V02max in the sedentary state: the HERITAGE family study. Med Sci Sports Exerc 1998;30:252–8.

397. Bouchard C, An P, Rice T, et al. Familial aggregation of V02max response to exercise training: results from the HERITAGE family study. J Appl Physiol 1999;87:1003–8.

398. National Association for Sport and Physical Education. Appropriate instructional practice guidelines for elementary school physical education. 3rd ed. Reston, VA: National Association for Sport and Physical Education; 2009. Available at http://www.cahperd.org/cms-assets/documents/ToolKit/NASPE_ApprroPrac/5287-207931.elementaryapproprac.pdf. Accessed July 15, 2011.

399. National Association for Sport and Physical Education. Appropriate instructional practice guidelines for middle school physical education. 3rd ed. Reston, VA: National Association for Sport and Physical Education; 2009. Available at http://www.cahperd.org/cms-assets/documents/ToolKit/NASPE_ApprroPrac/5289-666992.msapproprac.pdf. Accessed July 15, 2011.

400. National Association for Sport and Physical Education. Appropriate instructional practices for high school physical education. 3rd ed. Reston, VA: National Association for Sport and Physical Education; 2009. Available at http://www.cahperd.org/cms-assets/documents/ToolKit/NASPE_ApprroPrac/5288-573262.hsapproprac.pdf. Accessed July 15, 2011.

401. McKenzie TL, Feldman H, Woods SE, et al. Children's activity levels and lesson context during third-grade physical education. Res Q Exerc Sport 1995;66:184–93.

402. McKenzie T, Stone E, Feldman H, et al. Effects of the CATCH physical education intervention: teacher type and lesson location. Am J Prev Med 2001;21:101–9.

403. Fairclough S, Stratton G. Physical education makes you fit and healthy. Physical education's contribution to young people's physical activity levels. Health Educ Res 2005;20:14–23.

404. Scruggs PW, Beveridge SK, Eisenman PA, Watson DL, Shultz BB, Ransdell LB. Quantifying physical activity via pedometry in elementary physical education. Med Sci Sports Exerc 2003;35:1065–71.

405. Simons-Morton BG, Taylor WC, Snider SA, Huang IW, Fulton JE. Observed levels of elementary and middle school children's physical activity during physical education classes. Prev Med 1994;23:437–41.

406. van Beurden E, Barnett LM, Zask A, Dietrich UC, Brooks LO, Beard J. Can we skill and activate children through primary school physical education lessons? "Move it groove it"—a collaborative health promotion intervention. Prev Med 2003;36:493–501.

407. Baquet G, Berthoin S, Van PE. Are intensified physical education sessions able to elicit heart rate at a sufficient level to promote aerobic fitness in adolescents? Res Q Exerc Sport 2002;73:282–8.

408. Simons-Morton BG, Parcel G, Baranowski T, Forthofer R, O'Hara N. Promoting physical activity and a healthful diet among children: results of a school-based intervention study. Am J Public Health 1991;81:986–91.

409. Manios Y, Moschandreas J, Hatzis C, Kafatos A. Evaluation of a health and nutrition education program in primary school children of Crete over a three-year period. Prev Med 1999;28:149–59.

410. Vandongen R, Jenner DA, Thompson C, et al. A controlled evaluation of a fitness and nutrition intervention program on cardiovascular health in 10- to 12-year-old children. Prev Med 1995;24:9–22.

411. Dishman RK. Self-management strategies mediate self-efficacy and physical activity. Am J Prev Med 2005;29:10–8.

412. Shimon JM, Petlichkoff LM. Impact of pedometer use and self-regulation strategies on junior high school physical education students' daily step counts. J Phys Act Health 2009;6:178–84.

413. Motl RW, Dishman RK, Ward DS, et al. Comparison of barriers self-efficacy and perceived behavioral control for explaining physical activity across 1 year among adolescent girls. Health Psychol 2005;24:106–11.

414. Xiang P, Lee A. The development of self-perceptions of ability and achievement goals and their relations in physical education. Res Q Exerc Sport 1998;69:231–41.

415. Xiang P, McBride R, Guan J. Children's motivation in elementary physical education: a longitudinal study. Res Q Exerc Sport 2004;75:71–80.

416. Chase MA. Children's self-efficacy, motivational intentions, and attributions in physical education and sport. Res Q Exerc Sport 2001;72:47–54.

417. Papacharisis V, Goudas M. Perceptions about exercise and intrinsic motivation of students attending a health-related physical education program. Percept Mot Skills 2003;97:689–96.

418. Daley AJ, Buchana J. Aerobic dance and physical self-perceptions in female adolescents: some implications for physical education. Res Q Exerc Sport 1999;70:196–200.

419. Jago R, Baranowski T. Non-curricular approaches for increasing physical activity in youth: a review. Prev Med 2004;39:157–63.

420. National Association for Sport and Physical Education. Recess for elementary school students. Reston, VA: National Association for Sport and Physical Education; 2006. Available at http://www.aahperd.org/naspe/standards/upload/Recess-for-Elementary-School-Students-2006.pdf. Accessed July 15, 2011.

421. CDC. School health policies and programs study 2006 [unpublished data]. Atlanta, GA: US Department of Health and Human Services, CDC; 2009.

422. Ridgers ND, Stratton G, Fairclough SJ. Physical activity levels of children during school playtime. Sports Med 2006;36:359–71.

423. Ridgers ND, Stratton G, Fairclough SJ. Assessing physical activity during recess using accelerometry. Prev Med 2005;41:102–7.

424. Zask A, van Beurden E, Barnett L, Brooks LO, Dietrich UC. Active school playgrounds—myth or reality? Results of the "move it groove it" project. Prev Med 2001;33:402–8.

425. Burdette HL, Whitaker RC. Resurrecting free play in young children: looking beyond fitness and fatness to attention, affiliation, and affect. Arch Pediatr Adolesc Med 2005;159:46–50.

426. Sluckin A. Growing up in the playground: the social development of children. London, England: Routledge & Kegan Paul; 1981.

427. Barros RM, Silver EJ, Stein RE. School recess and group classroom behavior. Pediatr 2009;123:431–6.

428. Caterino MC, Polak ED. Effects of two types of activity on the performance of second-, third-, and fourth-grade students on a test of concentration. Percept Mot Skills 1999;89:245–8.

429. Pelligrini AD, Kato K, Blatchford P, Baines E. A short-term longitudinal study of children's playground games across the first year of school: implications for social competence and adjustment to school. Am Educ Res J 2002;39:991–1015.

430. Stratton G, Mullan E. The effect of multicolor playground markings on children's physical activity level during recess. Prev Med 2005;41:828–33.

431. Verstraete SJ, Cardon GM, De Clercq DL, De Bourdeaudhuij IM. Increasing children's physical activity levels during recess periods in elementary schools: the effects of providing game equipment. Eur J Pub Health 2006;23:1–5.

432. Robert Wood Johnson Foundation. Recess rules: why the undervalued playtime may be America's best investment for healthy kids and healthy schools. Princeton, NJ: Robert Wood Johnson Foundation; 2007. Available at http://www.rwjf.org/files/research/sports4kidsrecessreport.pdf. Accessed July 15, 2011.

433. Mahar MT, Murphy SK, Rowe DA, Golden J, Shields A, Raedeke TD. Effects of a classroom-based program on physical activity and on-task behavior. Medicine and science in sports and exercise 2006;38:2086–94.

434. Stewart JA, Dennison DA, Kohl HW, Doyle JA. Exercise level and energy expenditure in the TAKE 10! in-class physical activity program. J Sch Health 2004;74:397–400.

435. Kelder S, Hoelscher DM, Barroso CS, Walker JL, Cribb P, Hu S. The CATCH Kids Club: a pilot after-school study for improving elementary students' nutrition and physical activity. Public Health Nutr 2005;8:133–40.

436. Hellison D. Physical activity programs for underserved youth. J Sci Med Sport 2000;3:238–42.

437. Harrison PA, Gopalakrishnan N. Differences in behavior, psychological factors, and environmental factors associated with participation in school sports and other activities in adolescence. J Sch Health 2003;73:113–20.

438. Vilhjalmsson R, Kristjansdottir G. Gender differences in physical activity in older children and adolescents: the central role of organized sport. Soc Sci Med 2003;56:363–74.

439. Katzmarzyk PT, Malina R. Contribution of organized sports participation to estimated daily energy expenditure in youth. Pediatr Exerc Sci 2000;13:378–85.

440. Pate R, Trost S, Levin S, Dowda M. Sports participation and health-related behaviors among U.S. youth. Arch Pediatr Adolesc Med 2000;154:904–11.

441. Seefeldt V, Ewing ME. Youth sports in America. The President's Council on Physical Fitness and Sports Research Digest 1997;2:1–12.

442. Cooper AR, Page AS, Foster LJ, Qahwaji D. Commuting to school: are children who walk more physically active? Am J Prev Med 2003;25:273–6.

443. Cooper AR. Physical activity levels of children who walk, cycle, or are driven to school. Am J Prev Med 2005;29:179–84.

444. Tudor-Locke C, Neff LJ, Ainsworth BE, Addy CL, Popkin BM. Omission of active commuting to school and the prevalence of children's health-related physical activity levels: the Russian Longitudinal Monitoring Study. Child Care Health Dev 2002;28:507–12.

445. Alexander LM, Inchley J, Todd J, Currie D, Cooper AR, Currie C. The broader impact of walking to school among adolescents: seven day accelerometry based study. BMJ 2005;331:1061–2.

446. Sirard J, Riner WJ, McIver K, Pate R. Physical activity and active commuting to elementary school. Med Sci Sports Exerc 2005;37:2062–9.

447. Staunton CE, Hubsmith D, Kallins W. Promoting safe walking and bicycling to school: the Marin County success story. Am J Public Health 2003;93:1431–4.

448. CDC. Kids walk-to-school. A guide to promote walking to school. Atlanta, GA: US Department of Health and Human Services; 2006. Available at http://www.cdc.gov/nccdphp/dnpa/kidswalk/pdf/kidswalk.pdf. Accessed July 15, 2011.

449. Block ME, Klavina A, Flint W. Including students with severe, multiple disabilities in general physical education. JOPERD 2007;78:29–32.

450. Klavina A, Block ME. The effect of peer tutoring on interaction behaviors in inclusive physical education. Adapt Phys Activ Q 2008;25:132–58.

451. National Consortium for Physical Education and Recreation for Individuals with Disabilities. Adapted physical education national standards. 2nd ed. Champaign, IL: Human Kinetics; 2006.

452. Lohrmann DK, Wooley SF. Comprehensive school health education. In: Marx E, Wooley SF, eds. Health is academic. New York, NY: Teachers College Press; 1998:43–66.

453. Joint Committee on National Health Education Standards. National health education standards: achieving excellence. 2nd ed. Atlanta, GA: American Cancer Society; 2007.

454. Gold RS, Miner KR; 2000 Joint Committee on Health Education and Promotion Terminology. Report of the 2000 Joint Committee on Health Education and Promotion Terminology. J Sch Health 2002;72:3–7.

455. Kann L, Telljohann SK, Wooley S. Health education: results from the School Health Policies and Programs Study 2006. J Sch Health 2007;77:408–34.

456. Briggs M, Safaii S, Beall DL; American Dietetic Association; Society for Nutrition Education; American School Food Service Association. Position of the American Dietetic Association, Society for Nutrition Education, and American School Food Service Association—Nutrition services: an essential component of comprehensive school health programs. J Am Diet Assoc 2003;103:505–14.

457. Gortmaker SL, Peterson K, Wiecha J, et al. Reducing obesity via a school-based interdisciplinary intervention among youth: Planet Health. Arch Pediatr Adolesc Med 1999;153:409–18.

458. Moreno NP, Denk JP, Roberts JK, Tharp BZ, Bost M, Thompson WA. An approach to improving science knowledge about energy balance and nutrition among elementary- and middle-school students. Cell Biol Educ 2004;3:122–30.

459. Doak CM, Visscher TL, Renders CM, Seidell JC. The prevention of overweight and obesity in children and adolescents: a review of interventions and programmes. Obes Rev 2006;7:111–36.

460. Resnicow K, Davis M, Smith M, et al. How best to measure implementation of school health curricula: a comparison of three measures. Health Educ Res 1998;13:239–50.

461. Tomkins KO, Kamal KM, Chapman D. The West Virginia Health Education Assessment Project. J Sch Health 2005;75:193–8.

462. CDC. Health Education Curriculum Analysis Tool (HECAT). Atlanta, GA: US Department of Health and Human Services, CDC; 2007. Available at http://www.cdc.gov/healthyyouth/hecat/index.htm. Accessed July 15, 2011.

463. Popham WJ. Transformative assessment. Alexandria, VA: Association for Supervision and Curriculum Development; 2008.

464. Popham WJ. Instruction that measures up. Alexandria, VA: Association for Supervision and Curriculum Development; 2009.

465. Wiggins G, McTighe J. Understanding by design. 2nd ed. Alexandria VA: Association for Curriculum Development; 2005.

466. Marzano RJ, Pickering D, McTighe J. Assessing outcomes: performance assessment using dimensions of learning. Alexandria, VA: Association for Supervision and Curriculum Development; 1993.

467. Baranowski T. Gimme 5 fruit, juice, and vegetables for fun and health: outcome evaluation. Health Education & Behavior 2000;27:96–111.

468. Van Reusen K, Robinson J. Standards-based assessment in school health education. Education 1996;116:528–34.

469. Council of Chief State School Officers. State Collaborative on Assessment and Student Standards. Health Education Assessment Project (HEAP)—technical report. Washington, DC: Council of Chief State School Officers; 2000.

470. Lytle LA, Stone EJ, Nichaman MZ, et al. Changes in nutrient intakes of elementary school children following a school-based intervention: results from the CATCH Study. Prev Med 1996;25:465–77.

471. Nicklas TA, Johnson CC, Myers L, Farris RP, Cunningham A. Outcomes of a high school program to increase fruit and vegetable consumption: Gimme 5—a fresh nutrition concept for students. J Sch Health 1998;68:248–53.

472. Perry CL, Bishop DB, Taylor G, et al. Changing fruit and vegetable consumption among children: the 5-a-Day Power Plus program in St. Paul, Minnesota. Am J Public Health 1998;88:603–9.

473. Gortmaker SL, Cheung LW, Peterson KE, et al. Impact of a school-based interdisciplinary intervention on diet and physical activity among urban primary school children: eat well and keep moving. Arch Pediatr Adolesc Med 1999;153:975–83.

474. Harrell JS, Gansky SA, McMurray RG, Bangdiwala SI, Frauman AC, Bradley CB. School-based interventions improve heart health in children with multiple cardiovascular disease risk factors. Pediatrics 1998;102:371–80.

475. Manios Y, Kafatos A, Preventive Medicine and Nutrition Clinic University of Create Research Team. Health and nutrition education in primary schools in Crete: 10 years follow-up of serum lipids, physical activity and macronutrient intake. Br J Nutr 2006;95:568–75.

476. Kafatos I, Manios Y, Moschandreas J, Kafatos A. Health and nutrition education program in primary schools of Crete: changes in blood pressure over 10 years. Eur J Clin Nutr 2007;61:837–45.

477. Burke V, Thompson C, Taggart AC, et al. Differences in response to nutrition and fitness education programmes in relation to baseline levels of cardiovascular risk in 10- to 12-year-old children. J Hum Hypertens 1996;10(Suppl 3):S99–106.

478. Holcomb JD, Lira J, Kingery PM, Smith DW, Lane D, Goodway J. Evaluation of Jump Into Action: a program to reduce the risk of non-insulin dependent diabetes mellitus in school children on the Texas-Mexico border. J Sch Health 1998;68:282–8.

479. Trevino RP, Pugh JA, Hernandez AE, Menchaca VD, Ramirez RR, Mendoza M. Bienestar: a diabetes risk-factor prevention program. J Sch Health 1998;68:62–7.

480. Ritenbaugh C, Teufel-Shone NI, Aickin MG, et al. A lifestyle intervention improves plasma insulin levels among Native American high school youth. Prev Med 2003;36:309–19.

481. Shaw-Perry M, Horner C, Trevino RP, Sosa ET, Hernandez I, Bhardwaj A. NEEMA: A school-based diabetes risk prevention program designed for African-American Children. J Natl Med Assoc 2007;99:368–75.

482. Trevino RP, Yin Z, Hernandez A, Hale DE, Garcia OA, Mobley C. Impact of the bienestar school-based diabetes mellitus prevention program on fasting capillary glucose levels. Arch Pediatr Adolesc Med 2004;158:911–7.

483. Stang J, Taft Bayerl C, Flatt M, Associations Committee Positions Workgroup. Position of the American Dietetic Association: child and adolescent food and nutrition programs. J Am Diet Assoc 2006;106:1467–75.

484. Marcoux MF, Sallis JF, McKenzie TL, Marshall S, Armstrong CA, Goggin K. Process evaluation of a physical activity self-management program for children: SPARK. Psych Health 1999;14:659–77.

485. Allensworth DD. The research base for innovative practices in school health education at the secondary level. J Sch Health 1994;64:180–7.

486. Zahner L, Puder JJ, Roth R, et al. A school-based physical activity program to improve health and fitness in children aged 6–13 years ("Kinder-Sportstudie KISS"): study design of a randomized controlled trial. BMC Public Health 2006;6:147–59.

487. Bandura A. Social learning theory. Englewood Cliffs, NJ: Prentice Hall; 1997.

488. Shilts MS, Horowitz M, Townsend MS. Guided goal setting: effectiveness in a dietary and physical activity intervention with low-income adolescents. Int J Adolesc Med Health 2009;21:111–22.

489. Anderson AS, Porteous LE, Foster E, et al. The impact of a school-based nutrition education intervention on dietary intake and cognitive and attitudinal variables relating to fruits and vegetables. Pub Health Nutr 2005;8:650–6.

490. He M, Beynon C, Bouck MS, et al. Impact evaluation of the northern fruit and vegetable pilot programme—a clustered randomised controlled trial. Pub Health Nutr 2009;12:2199–208.

491. Dunton GF, Lagloire R, Robertson T. Using the RE-AIM framework to evaluate the statewide dissemination of a school-based physical activity and nutrition curriculum: "exercise your options." Am J Health Promot 2009;23:229–32.

492. Hoelscher DM, Evans A, Parcel GS, Kelder SH. Designing effective nutrition interventions for adolescents. J Am Diet Assoc 2002;102 (Suppl 3):S52–63.

493. Perez-Rodrigo C, Klepp KI, Yngve A, Sjostrom M, Stockley L, Aranceta J. The school setting: an opportunity for the implementation of dietary guidelines. Public Health Nutr 2001;4:717–24.

494. Perez-Rodrigo C, Aranceta J. School-based nutrition education: lessons learned and new perspectives. Public Health Nutr 2001;4:131–9.

495. Lavin AT. Comprehensive school health education: barriers and opportunities. J Sch Health 1993;63:24–7.

496. Rickard KA, Gallahue DL, Gruen GE, Tridle M, Bewley N, Steele K. The play approach to learning in the context of families and schools: an alternative paradigm for nutrition and fitness education in the 21st century. J Am Diet Assoc 1995;95:1121–6.

497. Contento IR, Kell DG, Keiley MK, Corcoran RD. A formative evaluation of the American Cancer Society changing the course nutrition education curriculum. J Sch Health 1992;62:411–6.

498. American Academy of Pediatrics Council on Sports Medicine and Fitness and Council on School Health. Active healthy living: prevention of childhood obesity through increased physical activity. Pediatrics 2006;117:1834–42.

499. Killen JD, Robinson TN. School-based research on health behavior change: the Stanford Adolescent Heart Health Program as a model for cardiovascular disease risk reduction [Chapter 4]. In: Rothkopf EZ, ed. Review of research in education. Washington, DC: American Education Research Association; 1988:171–200.

500. Howison D, Niedermyer F, Shortridge R. Field testing a fifth-grade nutrition education program designed to change food-selection behavior. J Nutr Educ 1988;20:82–6.

501. King AC, Saylor K, Foster S, et al. Promoting dietary change in adolescents: a school-based approach for modifying and maintaining healthful behavior. Am J Prev Med 1988;4:68–74.

502. Perry CL. Lessons from planet health. Arch Pediatr Adolesc Med 2005;159:292–3.

503. Long JD, Stevens KR. Using technology to promote self-efficacy for healthy eating in adolescents. J Nurs Scholarsh 2004;36:134–9.

504. Perez-Rodrigo C, Wind M, Hildonen C, et al. The pro children intervention: applying the intervention mapping protocol to develop a school-based fruit and vegetable promotion programme. Ann Nutr Metab 2005;49:267–77.

505. President's Council on Physical Fitness and Sports. The President's challenge. Washington, DC: President's Council on Physical Fitness and Sports; 2006.

506. Food and Nutrition Information Center. Database of food and nutrition software and multimedia programs [Database]. Beltsville, MD: US Department of Agriculture, National Agricultural Library, Food and Nutrition Information Center; 2005. Available at http://fnic.nal.usda.gov/nal_display/index.php?info_center=4&tax_level=1&tax_subject=253. Accessed July 15, 2011.

507. US Department of Agriculture. myPyramid.gov. [Internet site]. Alexandria, VA: US Department of Agriculture, Center for Nutrition Policy and Promotion; 2007. Available at http://www.choosemyplate.gov. Accessed July 15, 2011.

508. CDC. Healthy youth! Coordinated school health program. Atlanta, GA: US Department of Health and Human Services, CDC; 2008. Available at http://www.cdc.gov/healthyyouth/cshp. Accessed July 15, 2011.

509. American Academy of Pediatrics Council on School Health. Role of the school nurse in providing school health services. Pediatrics 2008; 121:1052–6.

510. Brener ND, Wheeler L, Wolfe LC, Vernon-Smiley M, Caldart-Olson L. Health services: results from the School Health Policies and Programs Study 2006. J Sch Health 2007;77:435–63.

511. National Association of School Nurses. Position statement: education, licensure, and certification of school nurses. Silver Spring, MD: National Association of School Nurses; 2002. Available at http://www.nasn.org/PolicyAdvocacy/PositionPapersandReports/NASNPositionStatementsArticleView/tabid/462/ArticleId/26/Education-Licensure-and-Certification-of-School-Nurses-Adopted-2002. Accessed July 15, 2011.

512. National Association of School Nurses. Resolution: access to a school nurse. Silver Spring, MD: National Association of School Nurses; 2003. Available at http://www.nasn.org/Portals/0/statements/resolutionaccess.pdf. Accessed July 15, 2011.

513. National Association of School Nurses. Position statement: overweight children and adolescents. Silver Spring, MD: National Association of School Nurses, Inc; 2002. Available at http://www.nasn.org/PolicyAdvocacy/PositionPapersandReports/NASNPositionStatementsFullView/tabid/462/smid/824/ArticleID/39/Default.aspx. Accessed July 15, 2011.

514. Vessey JA. Coordinated school health. Pediatr Nurs 2000;26:303–7.

515. National Association of School Nurses. Position Statement: role of the school nurse. Silver Spring, MD: National Association of School Nurses, Inc; 2002. Available at http://www.nasn.org/PolicyAdvocacy/PositionPapersandReports/NASNPositionStatementsFullView/tabid/462/ArticleId/87/Role-of-the-School-Nurse-Revised-2011. Accessed July 15, 2011.

516. Broussard BA, Sugarman JR, Bachman-Carter K, et al. Toward comprehensive obesity prevention programs in Native American communities. Obes Res 1995;3(Suppl 2):S289–97.

517. Small ML, Majer LS, Alensworth D, Farquhar BK, Kann L, Pateman B C. School health services. J Sch Health 1995;65:319–26.

518. Nihiser AJ, Lee SM, Wechsler H, et al. Body mass index measurement in schools. J Sch Health 2007;77:651–71.

519. American Academy of Pediatrics Committee on School Health. School health: policy & practice. 6th ed. Elk Grove, IL: American Academy of Pediatrics; 2004.

520. Davis MM, Gance-Cleveland B, Hassink S, Johnson R, Paradis G, Resnicow K. Recommendations for prevention of childhood obesity. Pediatrics 2007;120:S229–53.

521. National Association of School Nurses. S.C.O.P.E. School Nurse Childhood Obesity Prevention Education. Silver Spring, MD: National Association of School Nurses; 2009. Available at http://www.nasn.org/ContinuingEducation/LiveContinuingEducationPrograms/SCOPE. Accessed July 15, 2011.

522. American Academy of Pediatrics. Pediatric obesity clinical decision support chart. Elk Grove Village, IL: American Academy of Pediatrics; 2008.

523. Strong WB, Malina RM, Blimkie CJ, et al. Evidence based physical activity for school-age youth. J Pediatr 2005;146:732–7.

524. Taras HL, American Academy of Pediatrics Committee on School Health. School-based mental health services. Pediatrics 2004;113: 1839–45.

525. Griffiths LJ, Wolke D, Page AS, Horwood JP, the ALSPAC Study Team. Obesity and bullying: different effects for boys and girls. Arch Dis Child 2006;91:121–5.

526. Robinson S. Victimization of obese adolescents. J Sch Nurs 2006; 22:201–6.

527. Schwimmer JB, Burwinkle TM, Varni JW. Health-related quality of life of severely obese children and adolescents. JAMA 2003; 289:1813–9.

528. Sjoberg RL, Nilsson KW, Leppert J. Obesity, shame, and depression in school-aged children: A population-based study. Pediatrics 2005; 116:389–92.

529. Swallen KC, Reither EN, Haas SA, Meier AM. Overweight, obesity, and health-related quality of life among adolescents: The National Longitudinal Study of Adolescent Health. Pediatrics 2005; 115:340–7.

530. Killen JD, Taylor CB, Hayward C, et al. Pursuit of thinness and onset of eating disorder symptoms in a community sample of adolescent girls: a three-year prospective analysis. Int J Eat Disord 1994;16: 227–338.

531. Linde JA, Wall MM, Haines J, Neumark-Sztainer D. Predictors of initiation and persistence of unhealthy weight control behaviours in adolescents. Int J Behav Nutr Phys Act 2009;29:72.

532. Eaton DK, Lowry R, Brener ND, Galuska DA, Crosby AE. Associations of body mass index and perceived weight with suicide ideation and suicide attempts among U.S. high school students. Arch Pediatr Adolesc Med 2005;159:513–9.

533. Carmack BK. School NPs as advocates. Adv Nurse Pract 1997;5:74.

534. Nabors L, Troilette A, Nash T, Masiulis B. School nurse perceptions of barriers and supports for children with diabetes. J Sch Health 2005;75:119–24.

535. Rose BL, Mansour M, Kohake K. Building a partnership to evaluate school-linked health services: the Cincinnati School Health Demonstration Project. J Sch Health 2005;75:363–9.

536. Barrett Clayton J, Goodwin D, Kendrick O. Nursing, food service, and the child with diabetes. J Sch Nurs 2002;18:150–6.

537. Davidson M. Teaching teens to cope: coping skills training for adolescents with insulin-dependent diabetes mellitus. J Soc Pediatr Nurs 1997;2:65–72.

538. Erickson CD, Splett PL, Mullett SS, Heiman MB. The healthy learner model for student chronic condition management—part 1. J Sch Nurs 2006;22:310–8.

539. Spear BA, Barlow SE, Ervin C, et al. Recommendations for treatment of child and adolescent overweight and obesity. Pediatrics 2007;120 (Suppl 4):S254–88.

540. Nader PR, Kaczorowski J, Benioff S, Tonniges T, Schwartz D, Palfrey J. Education for community pediatrics. Clin Pediatr 2004;43:505–21.

541. Puskar KR, Weaver P, DeBlassio K. Nursing research in a school setting. J Sch Nurs 1994;10:8, 10–4.

542. Bradley BJ. The school nurse as health educator. J Sch Health 1997; 67:3–8.

543. Barlow SE, Dietz WH. Obesity evaluation and treatment: expert committee recommendations. J Pediatr 1998;102:E29. Epub Sept. 1, 1998. Available at http://pediatrics.aappublications.org/content/102/3/e29.full.html. Accessed July 15, 2011.

544. Himes JH, Dietz WH. Guidelines for overweight in adolescent preventive services: recommendations from an expert committee. The Expert Committee on Clinical Guidelines for Overweight in Adolescent Preventive Services. Am J Clin Nutr 1994;59:307–16.

545. Whitlock E, Williams S, Gold R, Smith P, Shipman S. Screening and interventions for childhood overweight: a summary of evidence for the U.S. Preventive Services Task Force. Pediatrics 2005;116:E125–44. Epub July 1, 2005. Available at http://pediatrics.aappublications.org/content/116/1/e125.short. Accessed July 15, 2011.

546. Howard KR. Childhood overweight: parental perceptions and readiness for change. J Sch Nurs 2007;23:73–9.

547. Downie J. The everyday realities of the multi-dimensional role of the high school community nurse. Aust J Adv Nurs 2002;19:15–24.

548. Lightfoot J. Working to keep school children healthy: the complementary roles of school staff and school nurses. J Public Health Med 2000;22:74–80.

549. National Association of School Nurses. The role of the school nurse in school based health centers: position statement. Silver Spring, MD: National Association of School Nurses, Inc.; 2001. Available at http://www.nasn.org/PolicyAdvocacy/PositionPapersandReports/NASNPositionStatementsArticleView/tabid/462/ArticleId/46/School-Based-Health-Centers-The-Role-of-the-School-Nurse-and-Revised-2011. Accessed July 19, 2011.

550. Barnes M. School based youth health nurses' role in assisting young people access health services in provincial, rural and remote areas of Queensland, Australia. Rural Remote Health 2004;4:279.

551. Barnett S, Duncan P, O'Connor KG. Pediatricians' response to the demand for school health programming. Pediatrics 1999;103:1–7.

552. Stang J, Story M, Kalina B. School-based weight management services: perceptions and practices of school nurses and administrators. Am J Health Promot 1997;11:183–5.

553. Moyers P, Bugle L, Jackson E. Perceptions of school nurses regarding obesity in school-age children. J School Nurs 2005;21:86–93.

554. Wehling Weepie A, McCarthy A. A healthy lifestyle program: promoting child health in schools. J Sch Nurs 2002;18:322–8.

555. Broussard L. School nursing: not just band-aids any more! J Spec Pediatr Nurs 2004;9:77–83.

556. Epstein JL, Sanders MG, Sheldon SB, et al. School, family, and community partnerships: your handbook for action. 3rd ed. Thousand Oaks, CA: Corwin Press; 2009.

557. Epstein J. School, family, and community partnerships: preparing educators and improving schools. Boulder, CO: Westview Press; 2001.

558. Henderson AL, Mara P. A new wave of evidence: the impact of school, family, and community connections on student achievement. Austin, TX: Southwest Educational Development Laboratory; 2002.

559. Gerne KM, Epstein JL. The power of partnerships: school, family, and community collaborations to improve children's health. RMC Health Educator 2004;4:1–7.

560. American Academy of Pediatrics. Family pediatrics: report of the task force on the family. Pediatrics 2003;111:1541–71.

561. Golan M, Weizman A. Familial approach to the treatment of childhood obesity: conceptual model. J Nutr Educ 2001;33:102–7.

562. Golan M, Crow S. Parents are key players in the prevention and treatment of weight-related problems. Nutr Rev 2004;62:39–50.

563. Baranowski T, Baranowski JC, Cullen KW, et al. The Fun, Food, and Fitness Project (FFFP): the Baylor GEMS pilot study. Ethn Dis 2003; 13(Suppl 1):S30–9.

564. Davis SM, Clay T, Smyth M, et al. Pathways curriculum and family interventions to promote healthful eating and physical activity in American Indian schoolchildren. Prev Med 2003;37(6 Pt 2):S24–34.

565. Fitzgibbon M, Stolley MR, Schiffer L, Van Horn L, KauferChristoffel K, Dyer A. Two-year follow-up results for Hip-Hop to Health Jr.: a randomized controlled trial for overweight prevention in preschool minority children. J Pediatr 2005;146:618–25.

566. Hopper CA, Gruber MB, Munoz KD, Herb RA. Effect of including parents in a school-based exercise and nutrition program for children. Res Q Exerc Sport 1992;63:315–21.

567. Hopper C, Munoz KD, Gruber MB, Nguyen KP. The effects of a family fitness program on the physical activity and nutrition behaviors of third-grade children. Res Q Exerc Sport 2005;76:130–9.

568. Nader PR, Sallis JF, Patterson T, et al. A family approach to cardiovascular risk reduction: results from the San Diego Family Health Project. Health Educ Q 1989;16:229–44.

569. Nader PR, Sellers DE, Johnson CC, et al. The effect of adult participation in a school-based family intervention to improve Children's diet and physical activity: the Child and Adolescent Trial for Cardiovascular Health. Prev Med 1996;25:455–64.

570. Perry CL, Luepker RV, Murray DV, et al. Parent involvement with children's health promotion: The Minnesota home team. Am J Public Health 1988;78:1156–60.

571. Ransdell LB, Taylor A, Oakland D, Schmidt J, Moyer-Mileur L, Shultz B. Daughters and mothers exercising together: effects of home- and community-based programs. Med Sci Sports Exerc 2003;35:286–96.

572. Steckler A, Ethelbah B, Martin CJ, et al. Pathways process evaluation results: a school-based prevention trial to promote healthful diet and physical activity in American Indian third, fourth, and fifth grade students. Prev Med 2003;37(6 Pt 2):S80–90.

573. Stolley MR, Fitzgibbon ML. Effects of an obesity prevention program on the eating behavior of African American mothers and daughters. Health Educ Behav 1997;24:152–64.

574. Story M, Sherwood NE, Himes JH, et al. An after-school obesity prevention program for African-American girls: The Minnesota GEMS pilot study. Ethn Dis 2003;13(Suppl 1):S54–64.

575. Trevino RP, Hernandez AE, Yin Z, Garcia OA, Hernandez I. Effect of the Bienestar Health Program on physical fitness in low-income Mexican American children. Hisp J Behav Sci 2005;27:120–32.

576. Beech BM, Klesges RC, Kumanyika SK, et al. Child- and parent-targeted interventions: the Memphis GEMS pilot study. Ethn Dis 2003;13(Suppl 1):S40–53.

577. Weeks K, Levy SR, Gordon AK, Handler A, Perhats C, Flay BR. Does parental involvement make a difference? The impact of parent interactive activities on students in a school-based AIDS prevention program. AIDS Educ Prev 1997;9(Suppl 1):90–106.

578. Golan M, Crow S. Targeting parents exclusively in the treatment of childhood obesity: long-term results. Obes Res 2004;12.

579. Golan M, Fainaru M, Weizman A. Role of behaviour modification in the treatment of childhood obesity with the parents as the exclusive agents of change. Int J Obes Relat Metab Disord 1998;22:1217–24.

580. McGarvey E, Keller A, Forrester M, Williams E, Seward D, Suttle DE. Feasibility and benefits of a parent-focused preschool child obesity intervention. Am J Public Health 2004;94:1490–5.

581. McLean N, Griffin S, Toney K, Hardeman W. Family involvement in weight control, weight maintenance and weight-loss interventions: a systematic review of randomised trials. Int J Obes Relat Metab Disord 2003;27:987–1005.

582. Epstein LH, Voloski A, Wing RR, McCurley J. Ten-year outcomes of behavioral family-based treatment for childhood obesity. Health Psych 1994;13:373–83.

583. Coleman KJ, Tiller CL, Sanchez J, et al. Prevention of the epidemic increase in child risk of overweight in low-income schools: the El Paso coordinated approach to child health. Arch Pediatr Adolesc Med 2005;159:217–24.

584. Elder JP, Campbell NR, Candelaria JI, et al. Project salsa: development and institutionalization of a nutritional health promotion project in a Latino community. Am J Health Promot 1998;12:391–401.

585. Good TL, Wiley AR, Thomas RE, et al. Bridging the gap between schools and community: organizing for family involvement in a low-income neighborhood. JEPC 1997;8:277–96.

586. Landis SE, Janes CL. The Claxton Elementary School Health Program: merging perceptions and behaviors to identify problems. J Sch Health 1995;65:250–4.

587. Kakli Z, Kreider H, Little P, Buck T, Coffey M. Focus on families! How to build and support family-centered practices in after school. Boston, MA: United Way of Massachusetts Bay; Harvard Family Research Project; Build the Out-of-School Time Network; 2006. Available at http://www.hfrp.org/family-involvement/publications-resources/focus-on-families!-how-to-build-and-support-family-centered-practices-in-after-school. Accessed July 22, 2011.

588. Pate RR, Saunders RP, Ward DS, Felton G, Trost SG, Dowda M. Evaluation of a community-based intervention to promote physical activity in youth: lessons from Active Winners. Am J Health Promot 2003;17:171–82.

589. Economos CD, Hyatt RR, Goldberg JP, et al. A community intervention reduces BMI z-score in children: Shape Up Somerville first year results. Obesity Res 2007;15:1325–36.

590. Pentz MA. The school-community interface in comprehensive school health education. In: Allensworth D, Lawson E, Nicholson L, Wyche J, eds. Schools and health. Washington, DC: National Academy Press; 1997. 305–36.

591. Margolis PA, Stevens R, Bordley C, et al. From concept to application: the impact of a community-wide intervention to improve the delivery of preventive services to children. Pediatrics 2001;108:42–52.

592. Policy Leadership for Active Youth. Addressing overweight: interventions tailored to the rural south. Atlanta, GA: Georgia State University; 2005.

593. Michael S, Dittus P, Epstein J. Family and community involvement in schools: results from the school health policies and programs study 2006. J Sch Health 2007;77:567–79.

594. Gittelsohn J, Davis SM, Steckler A, et al. Pathways: lessons learned and future directions for school-based interventions among American Indians. Prev Med 2003;37(6 Pt 2):S107–12.

595. Lytle LA, Kubik MY, Perry C, Story M, Birnbaum AS, Murray DM. Influencing healthful food choices in school and home environments: results from the TEENS study. Prev Med 2006;43:8–13.

596. Cohen L, Baer N, Satterwhite P. Developing effective coalitions: an eight step guide. In: Wurzbach J, ed. Community health education and promotion: a guide to program design and evaluation. 2nd ed. Gaithersburg, MD: Aspen Publishers Inc; 2002:144–61.

597. Felton G, Saunders RP, Ward DS, Dishman RK, Dowda M, Pate RR. Promoting physical activity in girls: a case study of one school's success. J Sch Health 2005;75:57–62.

598. Lopez R, Campbell R, Jennings J. The Boston schoolyard initiative: a public-private partnership for rebuilding urban play space. J Health Polit Policy Law 2008;33:617–38.

599. Story M, Nanney MS, Schwartz MB. Schools and obesity prevention: creating school environments and policies to promote healthy eating and physical activity. Milbank Q 2009;87:71–100.

600. White House Task Force on Childhood Obesity. Childhood Obesity Task Force unveils action plan. Solving the problem of childhood obesity within a generation: report to the president. Washington, DC: Executive Office of the President of the United States; 2010. Available at http://www.whitehouse.gov/the-press-office/childhood-obesity-task-force-unveils-action-plan-solving-problem-childhood-obesity-. Accessed July 22, 2011.

601. National Policy and Legal Analysis Network to Prevent Childhood Obesity. Joint use agreement 3: opening school facilities for use during non-school hours and authorizing third parties to operate programs. Oakland, CA: National Policy and Legal Analysis Network to Prevent Childhood Obesity; 2009. Available at http://www.whitehouse.gov/the-press-office/childhood-obesity-task-force-unveils-action-plan-solving-problem-childhood-obesity-. Accessed July 22, 2011.

602. Fothergill K, Ballard E. The school-linked health center: a promising model of community-based care for adolescents. J Adolesc Health 1998;23:29–38.

603. Juhn G, Tang J, Piessens P, Grant U, Johnson N, Murray H. Community learning: the reach for health nursing program-middle school collaboration. J Nurs Educ 1999;38:215–21.

604. Strelow JS, Larsen JS, Sallis JF, Conway TL, Powers HS, McKenzie TL. Factors influencing the performance of volunteers who provide physical activity in middle schools. J Sch Health 2002;72:147–51.

605. Agron P, Berends V, Cole N, Gooley J, Hawksworth K, Martinez N. Engaging parents and stakeholders in school wellness: formative research report. Los Angeles, CA: The California Endowment; 2008. Available at http://www.californiaprojectlean.org/docuserfiles//Parent%20Formative%20Research%20Report.pdf. Accessed July 22, 2011.

606. Pate RR, O'Neill JR. After-school interventions to increase physical activity among youth. Br J Sports Med 2009;43:14–8.

607. Robinson TN, Killen JD, Kraemer HC, et al. Dance and reducing television viewing to prevent weight gain in African-American girls: the Stanford GEMS pilot study. Ethn Dis 2003;13(Suppl 1): S65–77.

608. Marschall M. Parent involvement and educational outcomes for Latino students. Rev Policy Res 2006;23:1053–76.

609. Davis SM, Going SB, Helitzer DL, et al. Pathways: a culturally appropriate obesity-prevention program for American Indian schoolchildren. Am J Clin Nutr 1999;69(Suppl 4):S796–802.

610. Snyder TD, Tan AG. Digest of education statistics, 2004. NCES 2006005. Washington, DC: National Center for Education Statistics; 2005. Available at http://nces.ed.gov/pubsearch/pubsinfo.asp?pubid=2006005. Accessed July 22, 2011.

611. Aldana SG. Financial impact of health promotion programs: a review of the literature. Am J Health Promot 2001;15:296–320.

612. Davis L, Loyo K, Glowka A, et al. A comprehensive worksite wellness program in Austin, Texas: partnership between Steps to a Healthier Austin and Capital Metropolitan Transportation Authority. Prev Chronic Dis 2009;6:A60.

613. Wisconsin Department of Health and Family Services, Division of Public Health, Nutrition and Physical Activity Program, Wisconsin Partnership for Activity and Nutrition. Wisconsin worksite resource kit to prevent obesity and related chronic diseases. Madison, WI: Wisconsin Department of Health and Family Services; 2007.

614. Partnership for Prevention. Healthy workforce 2010: an essential health promotion sourcebook for employers large and small. Washington, DC: Partnership for Prevention; 2001. Available at http://www.acsworkplacesolutions.com/documents/Healthy_Workforce_2010.pdf. Accessed July 22, 2011.

615. Aldana SG, Pronk NP. Health promotion programs, modifiable health risks, and employee absenteeism. J Occup Environ Med 2001;43:36–46.

616. Allegrante JP, Michela JL. Impact of a school-based workplace health promotion program on morale of inner-city teachers. J Sch Health 1990;60:25–8.

617. Blair SN, Collingwood TR, Reynolds K, Smith M, Hagan RD, Sterling CL. Health promotion for educators: impact on health behaviors, satisfaction, and general well-being. Am J Public Health 1984;74: 147–9.

618. Cullen KW, Baranowski T, Herbert D, deMoor C, Hearn MD, Resnicow K. Influence of school organizational characteristics on the outcomes of a school health promotion program. J Sch Health 1999; 69:376–80.

619. Galemore CA. Initiation of a school employee wellness program: applying the comprehensive health education model. J Sch Nurs 2000; 16:39–46.

620. Galemore CA. Worksite wellness in the school setting. J Sch Nurs 2000; 16:42–5.

621. Galaif ER, Sussman S, Bundek N. The relations of school staff smokers' attitudes about modeling smoking behavior in students and their receptivity to no-smoking policy. J Drug Educ 1996;26:313–22.

622. Kumar R, O'Malley PM, Johnston LD, Schulenberg JE, Gachman JG. Effects of school-level norms on student substance use. Prev Sci 2002;3:105–24.

623. Trinidad DR, Gilpin EA, Pierce JP. Compliance and support for smoke-free school policies. Health Educ Res 2005;20:466–75.

624. Eaton DK, Marx E, Bowie SE. Faculty and staff health promotion: results from the School Health Policies and Programs Study 2006. J Sch Health 2007;77:557–66.

625. Directors of Health Promotion and Education. School employee wellness: a guide for protecting the assets of our nation's schools. Washington, DC: Directors of Health Promotion and Education; 2007. Available at http://www.whf.org/documents/coordinated-school-health-docs/School%20Employee%20Wellness%20-%20Establishing%20Wellness.pdf. Accessed July 22, 2011.

626. Engbers LH, van Poppel MN, Chin AP, van Mechelen W. Worksite health promotion programs with environmental changes: a systematic review. Am J Prev Med 2005;29:61–70.

627. Marshall AL, Owen N, Bauman A. Mediated approaches for influencing physical activity: update of the evidence on mass media, print, telephone and website delivery of interventions. J Sci Med Sport 2004;7:74–80.

628. Brissette I, Fisher B, Spicer DA, King L. Worksite characteristics and environmental and policy supports for cardiovascular disease prevention in New York State. Prev Chronic Dis 2008;5:A37.

629. Hawkins C, O'Garro MA, Wimsett K. Engaging employers to develop healthy workplaces: the WorkWell initiative of Steps to a Healthier Washington in Thurston County. Prev Chronic Dis 2009;6:A61.

630. Oldenburg B, Sallis JF, Harris D, Owen N. Checklist of health promotion environments at worksites (CHEW): development and measurement characteristics. Am J Health Promot 2002;16:288–99.

631. Zunker C, Cox TL, Wingo BC, Knight B, Jefferson WK, Ard JD. Using formative research to develop a worksite health promotion program for African American women. Women Health 2008;48: 189–207.

632. Bearden JB. Maine school district goes all out for employee wellness. School Business Affairs 2005;71:26–7.

633. CDC. Public health strategies for preventing and controlling overweight and obesity in school and worksite settings. A report on recommendations of the Task Force on Community Preventive Services. MMWR 2005; 54:1–12.

634. Taylor WC. Transforming work breaks to promote health. Am J Prev Med 2005;29:461–5.

635. Yancey A, McCarthy W, Taylor W, et al. The Los Angeles Lift Off: a sociocultural environmental change intervention to integrate physical activity into the workplace. Prev Med 2004;38:848–56.

636. Chan CB, Ryan DA, Tudor-Locke C. Health benefits of a pedometer-based physical activity intervention in sedentary workers. Prev Med 2004;39:1215–22.

637. Matson-Koffman DM, Brownstein JN, Neiner JA, Greaney ML. A site-specific literature review of policy and environmental interventions that promote physical activity and nutrition for cardiovascular health: what works? Am J Health Promot 2005;19:167–93.

638. Patterson R, Kristal AR, Biener L, et al. Durability and diffusion of the nutrition intervention in the Working Well Trial. Prev Med 1998; 27:668–73.

639. White JL, Ransdell LB. Worksite intervention model for facilitating changes in physical activity, fitness, and psychological parameteres. Percept Mot Skills 2003;97:461–6.

640. Auld G, Romaniello C, Heimendinger J, Hambidge C, Hambidge M. Outcomes from a school-based nutrition education program using resource teachers and cross-disciplinary models. J Nutr Educ 1998; 30:268–80.

641. Davis K, Burgeson CR, Brener ND, McManus T, Wechsler H. The relationship between qualified personnel and self-reported implementation of recommended physical education practices and programs in U.S. schools. Res Q Exerc Sport 2005;76:202–11.

642. Fulkerson JA, French SA, Story MA, Syder P, Paddock M. Foodservice staff perceptions of their influence on student food choices. J Am Diet Assoc 2002;102:97–9.

643. Dwyer JJ, Allison KR, Barrera M, Hansen B, Goldenberg E, Boutilier MA. Teachers' perspective on barriers to implementing physical activity curriculum guidelines for school children in Toronto. Can J Public Health 2003;94:448–52.

644. Kelder SH, Mitchell PD, McKenzie TL, et al. Long-term implementation of the CATCH physical education program. Health Educ Behav 2003;30:463–75.

645. Kulinna PH, Silverman S. Teachers' attitudes toward teaching physical activity and fitness. Res Q Exerc Sport 2000;71:80–4.

646. Davis M, Baranowski T, Resnicow K, et al. Gimme 5 fruit and vegetables for fun and health: process evaluation. Health Educ Behav 2000;27:167–76.

647. National Association for Sport and Physical Education. National standards for beginning physical education teachers. 2nd ed. Reston, VA: National Association for Sport and Physical Education; 2009.

648. National Association for Sport and Physical Education. Opportunity to learn standards for elementary school physical education. Reston, VA: National Association for Sport and Physical Education; 2000.

649. National Association for Sport and Physical Education. Opportunity to learn standards for high school physical education. Reston, VA: National Association for Sport and Physical Education; 2004.

650. National Association for Sport and Physical Education. Opportunity to learn standards for middle school physical education. Reston, VA: National Association for Sport and Physical Education; 2004.

651. Kealey KA, Peterson AV Jr, Gaul MA, Dinh KT. Teacher training as a behavior change process: principles and results from a longitudinal study. Health Educ Behav 2000;27:64–81.

652. Pateman B, Grunbaum JA, Kann L. Voices from the field—a qualitative analysis of classroom, school, district, and state health education policies and programs. J Sch Health 1999;69:258–63.

653. Stang J, Story M, Kalina B. Nutrition education in Minnesota public schools: perceptions and practices of teachers. J Nutr Educ 1998;30:396–404.

654. American Association for Health Education. AAHE/NCATE health education standards and key elements. Reston, VA: American Association for Health Education; 2001.

655. Coalition of National Health Education Organizations. The health education profession in the 21st century: setting the stage. J Sch Health 1996;66:291–8.

656. Cater JM, Carr DH. Competencies, knowledge, and skills of effective school nutrition managers. R-66-03. University, MS: National Food Service Management Institute; 2004.

657. Rainville AJ, Carr DH. Competencies, knowledge, and skill statements for district school nutrition directors/supervisors. R-50-01. University, MS, National Food Service Management Institute; 2001.

658. Gross S, Cinelli B. Coordinated school health program and dietetics professionals: partners in promoting healthful eating. J Am Diet Assoc 2004;104:793–8.

659. Wei RC, Darling-Hammond L, Andree A, Richardson N, Orphanos S. Professional learning in the learning profession: a status report on teacher development in the United States and abroad. Dallas, TX: National Staff Development Council; 2009. Available at http://www.nsdc.org/news/NSDCstudy2009.pdf. Accessed July 22, 2011.

660. National Association for Sport and Physical Education. Physical activity and fitness recommendations for physical activity professionals. Reston, VA: National Association for Sport and Physical Education; 2002.

661. Wiecha JL, El Ayadi AM, Fuemmeler BF, et al. Diffusion of an integrated health education program in an urban school system: planet health. J Pediatr Psychol 2004;29:467–74.

662. Weiler R, Pigg RM Jr. An evaluation of client satisfaction with training programs and technical assistance provided by Florida's Coordinated School Health Program Office. J Sch Health 2000;70:361–7.

663. McKenzie TL, Sallis JF, Kolody B, Faucette FN. Long-term effects of a physical education curriculum and staff development program: SPARK. Res Q Exerc Sport 1997;68:280–91.

664. Fairclough S, Stratton G. Improving health-enhancing physical activity in girls' physical education. Health Educ Res 2005;20:448–57.

665. State of Michigan Department of Education. Fully qualified teachers of health education. Lansing, MI: State of Michigan Department of Education; 2005.

666. Peregrin T. Take 10! Classroom-based program fights obesity by getting kids out of their seats. J Am Diet Assoc 2001;101:1409.

667. Edmundson E, Parcel GS, Feldman HA, et al. The effects of the Child and Adolescent Trial for Cardiovascular Health upon psychosocial determinants of diet and physical activity behavior. Prev Med 1996;25:442–54.

668. Johnson CC, Galati T, Pedersen S, Smyth M, Parcel GS. Maintenance of the classroom health education curricula: results from the CATCH-ON study. Health Educ Beh 2003;30:476–88.

669. Geiger BF, Petri CJ, Myers O, et al. Using technology to teach health: a collaborative pilot project in Alabama. J Sch Health 2002;72:401–7.

670. Jones Everett S, Brenner N, McManus T. The relationship between staff development and health instruction in schools in the United States. J health Educ 2004;35:2.

671. Bauer KW, Patel A, Prokop LA, Austin Bryn S. Swimming upstream: faculty and staff members from urban middle schools in low-income communities describe their experience implementing nutrition and physical activity initiatives. Prev Chronic Dis 2006;3:A37–45.

672. Sullivan K, Harper M, West CK. Professional development needs reported by school food service directors and recommendations for meeting directors' needs. Oxford, MS: National Food Service Management Institute; 2000.

673. Osganian SK, Ebzery MK, Montgomery DH, et al. Changes in the nutrient content of school lunches: results from the CATCH Eat Smart Food service Intervention. Prev Med 1996;25:400–12.

674. Halpern R. After-school programs for low-income children: promise and challenges. Future child 1999;9:81–95.

675. Neighbors M, Barta K. School nurse summer institute: a model for professional development. J Sch Nurs 2004;20:134–8.

676. Saaranen T, Tossavainen K, Turunen H. School staff members' and occupational health nurses' evaluation of the promotion of occupational well-being—with good planning to better practice. J Interprof Care 2005;19:465–79.

677. Brener ND, Weist M, Adelman H, Taylor L, Vernon-Smiley M. Mental health and social services: results from the School Health Policies and Programs Study 2006. J Sch Health 2007;77:464–85.

678. US Department of Agriculture, Food and Nutrition Service. The power of choice: helping youth make healthy eating and fitness decisions. Washington, DC: US Department of Agriculture; 2003.

679. Libman S. Adult participation in youth sports. A developmental perspective. Child Adolesc Psychiatr Clin N Am 1998;7:725–44.

680. Wiersma LD, Sherman CP. Volunteer youth sport coaches' perspectives of coaching education/certification and parental codes of conduct. Res Q Exerc Sport 2005;76:324–38.

Appendix A

Summary of *School Health Guidelines to Promote Healthy Eating and Physical Activity*

Guideline 1: Use a coordinated approach to develop, implement, and evaluate healthy eating and physical activity policies and practices

- Coordinate healthy eating and physical activity policies and practices through a school health council and school health coordinator.
- Assess healthy eating and physical activity policies and practices.
- Use a systematic approach to develop, implement, and monitor healthy eating and physical activity policies.
- Evaluate healthy eating and physical activity policies and practices.

Guideline 2: Establish school environments that support healthy eating and physical activity

- Provide access to healthy foods and physical activity opportunities and to safe spaces, facilities, and equipment for healthy eating and physical activity.
- Establish a climate that encourages and does not stigmatize healthy eating and physical activity.
- Create a school environment that encourages a healthy body image, shape, and size among all students and staff members, is accepting of diverse abilities, and does not tolerate weight-based teasing.

Guideline 3: Provide a quality school meal program and ensure that students have only appealing, healthy food and beverage choices offered outside of the school meal program

- Promote access to and participation in school meals.
- Provide nutritious and appealing school meals that comply with the *Dietary Guidelines for Americans*.
- Ensure that all foods and beverages sold or served outside of school meal programs are nutritious and appealing.

Guideline 4: Implement a comprehensive physical activity program with quality physical education as the cornerstone

- Require students in grades K–12 to participate in daily physical education that uses a planned and sequential curriculum and instructional practices that are consistent with national or state standards for physical education.
- Provide a substantial percentage of each student's recommended daily amount of physical activity in physical education class.
- Use instructional strategies in physical education that enhance students' behavioral skills, confidence in their abilities, and desire to adopt and maintain a physically active lifestyle.
- Provide ample opportunities for all students to engage in physical activity outside of physical education class.
- Ensure that physical education and other physical activity programs meet the needs and interests of all students.

Guideline 5: Implement health education that provides students with the knowledge, attitudes, skills, and experiences needed for lifelong healthy eating and physical activity

- Require health education from prekindergarten through grade 12.
- Implement a planned and sequential health education curriculum that is culturally and developmentally appropriate, addresses a clear set of behavioral outcomes that promote healthy eating and physical activity, and is based on national standards.
- Use curricula that are consistent with scientific evidence of effectiveness in helping students improve healthy eating and physical activity behaviors.
- Use classroom instructional methods and strategies that are interactive, engage all students, and are relevant to their daily lives and experiences.

Guideline 6: Provide students with health, mental health, and social services to address healthy eating, physical activity, and related chronic disease prevention

- Assess student needs related to physical activity, nutrition, and obesity, and provide counseling and other services to meet those needs.

- Ensure students have access to needed health, mental health, and social services.

- Provide leadership in advocacy and coordination of effective school physical activity and nutrition policies and practices.

Guideline 7: Partner with families and community members in the development and implementation of healthy eating and physical activity policies, practices, and programs

- Encourage communication among schools, families and community members to promote adoption of healthy eating and physical activity behaviors among students.

- Involve families and community members on the school health council.

- Develop and implement strategies for motivating families to participate in school-based programs and activities that promote healthy eating and physical activity.

- Access community resources to help provide healthy eating and physical activity opportunities for students.

- Demonstrate cultural awareness in healthy eating and physical activity practices throughout the school.

Guideline 8: Provide a school employee wellness program that includes healthy eating and physical activity services for all school staff members

- Gather data and information to determine the nutrition and physical activity needs of school staff members and assess the availability of existing school employee wellness activities and resources.

- Encourage administrative support for and staff involvement in school employee wellness.

- Develop, implement, and evaluate healthy eating and physical activity programs for all school employees.

Guideline 9: Employ qualified persons, and provide professional development opportunities for physical education, health education, nutrition services, and health, mental health, and social services staff members, as well as staff members who supervise recess, cafeteria time, and out-of-school–time programs

- Require the hiring of physical education teachers, health education teachers, and nutrition services staff members who are certified and appropriately prepared to deliver quality instruction, programs, and practices.

- Provide school staff members with annual professional development opportunities to deliver quality physical education, health education, and nutrition services.

- Provide annual professional development opportunities for school health, mental health, and social services staff members and staff members who lead or supervise out-of-school–time programs, recess, and cafeteria time.

Appendix B

Healthy People 2020 Objectives for Healthy Eating and Physical Activity Among Children and Adolescents

Nutrition and Weight Status (NWS) Objectives

NWS 2: Increase the proportion of schools that offer nutritious foods and beverages outside of school meals.

  NWS 2.1: Increase the proportion of schools that do not sell or offer calorically sweetened beverages to students.

  NWS 2.2: Increase the proportion of school districts that require schools to make fruits or vegetables available whenever other food is offered or sold.

NWS 10: Reduce the proportion of children and adolescents who are considered obese.

NWS 11: (Developmental) Prevent inappropriate weight gain in youths and adults.

NWS 14: Increase the contribution of fruits to the diets of the population aged ≥2 years.

NWS 15: Increase the variety and contribution of vegetables to the diets of the population aged ≥2 years.

  NWS 15.2: Increase the contribution of dark green vegetables, orange vegetables, and legumes to the diets of the population aged ≥2 years.

NWS 16: Increase the contribution of whole grains to the diets of the population aged ≥2 years.

NWS 17: Reduce consumption of calories from solid fats and added sugars in the population ≥2 years.

NWS 18: Reduce consumption of saturated fat in the population aged ≥2 years.

NWS 19: Reduce consumption of sodium in the population aged ≥2 years.

NWS 20: Increase consumption of calcium in the population aged ≥2 years.

NWS 21: Reduce iron deficiency among young children and females of childbearing age.

Physical Activity (PA) Objectives

PA 3: Increase the proportion of adolescents who meet current federal physical activity guidelines for aerobic physical activity and for muscle-strengthening activity.

PA 4: Increase the proportion of the nation's public and private schools that require daily physical education for all students.

PA 5: Increase the proportion of adolescents who participated in daily school physical education.

PA 6: Increase regularly scheduled elementary school recess in the United States.

  PA 6.1: Increase the number of states that require regularly scheduled elementary school recess.

  PA 6.2: Increase the proportion of school districts that require regularly scheduled elementary school recess.

PA 7: Increase the proportion of school districts that require or recommend elementary school recess for an appropriate period of time.

PA 8: Increase the proportion of children and adolescents who do not exceed recommended limits for screen time.

  PA 8.2: Increase the proportion of children and adolescents aged 2 years through 12th grade who view television, videos, or play video games for no more than 2 hours a day.

PA 10: Increase the proportion of the nation's public and private schools that provide access to their physical activity spaces and facilities for all persons outside of normal school hours (e.g., before and after the school day, on weekends, and during summer and other vacations).

PA 13: Increase the proportion of trips made by walking.

  PA 13.2: Children and adolescents aged 5–15 years, trips to school of ≤1 mile.

PA 14: Increase the proportion of trips made by bicycling.

  PA 14.2: Children and adolescents aged 5–15 years, trips to school of ≤2 miles.

Early and Middle Childhood (EMC) Objectives

EMC 4:   Increase the proportion of elementary, middle, and senior high schools that require school health education.

EMC 4.1:   Increase the proportion of schools that require newly hired staff who teach required health education to have undergraduate or graduate training in health education.

EMC 4.2:   Increase the proportion of schools that require newly hired staff who teach required health instruction to be certified, licensed, or endorsed by the state in health education.

EMC 4.4:   Increase the proportion of required health education classes or courses with a teacher who has had professional development related to teaching personal and social skills for behavior change within the past 2 years.

Educational and Community-Based Programs (ECBP) Objectives

ECBP 2:   Increase the proportion of elementary, middle, and senior high schools that provide comprehensive school health education to prevent health problems in:

ECBP 2.8:   Unhealthy dietary patterns.

ECBP 2.9:   Inadequate physical activity.

ECBP 3:   Increase the proportion of elementary, middle, and senior high schools that have health education goals or objectives that address the knowledge and skills articulated in the National Health Education Standards (high school, middle, and elementary).

ECBP 4:   Increase the proportion of elementary, middle, and senior high schools that provide school health education to promote personal health and wellness in the following areas:

ECBP 4.3:   Growth and development.

ECBP 5:   Increase the proportion of the nation's elementary, middle, and senior high schools that have a full-time registered school nurse-student ratio of at least 1:750.

ECBP 8:   (Developmental) Increase the proportion of worksites that offer an employee health promotion program to their employees.

Technical Advisors for *School Health Guidelines to Promote Healthy Eating and Physical Activity*

Individual Advisors

Lisa C. Barrios, DrPH, Gema G. Dumitru, MD, Marci F. Hertz, MSEd, Sarah M. Lee, PhD, Caitlin L. Merlo, MPH, Allison J. Nihiser, MPH, Leah Robin, PhD, Terrence P. O'Toole, PhD, Howell Wechsler, EdD, CDC, Atlanta, Georgia; Mara Galic, MHSc, Columbus Technologies, Atlanta, Georgia; Michael W. Beets, PhD, University of South Carolina, Columbia, South Carolina; Glenn Flores, MD, University of Texas Southwestern Medical Center, Dallas, Texas; Deanna M. Hoelscher, PhD, University of Texas, Houston, Texas; Leslie A. Lytle, PhD, University of Minnesota, Minneapolis, Minnesota; Mary McKenna, PhD, University of New Brunswick, Fredericton, New Brunswick, Canada; Russell R. Pate, PhD, University of South Carolina, Columbia, South Carolina; Claudia K. Probart, PhD, The Pennsylvania State University, University Park, Pennsylvania; Marlene B. Schwartz, PhD, Yale Rudd Center for Food Policy and Obesity, Yale University, New Haven, Connecticut; Mary Story, PhD, University of Minnesota, Minneapolis, Minnesota; Howard Taras, MD, University of California San Diego, La Jolla, California; Wendell C. Taylor, PhD, University of Texas, Houston, Texas; Stewart G. Trost, PhD, Oregon State University, Corvallis, Oregon; Diane Stanton Ward, EdD, University of North Carolina, Chapel Hill, North Carolina; Greg J. Welk, PhD, Iowa State University, Ames, Iowa.

Federal and State Agencies

President's Council on Fitness, Sports and Nutrition, U.S. Department of Health and Human Services, Rockville, Maryland; Food and Nutrition Service, U.S. Department of Agriculture, Alexandria, Virginia; Office of Safe and Drug-Free Schools, U.S. Department of Education, Washington, DC; Arizona Department of Education, Phoenix, Arizona; Colorado Department of Education, Denver, Colorado; Massachusetts Department of Elementary and Secondary Education, Malden, Massachusetts; Michigan Department of Education, Lansing, Michigan; Wisconsin Department of Public Instruction, Madison, Wisconsin.

National and State Organizations

Achievability, Philadelphia, Pennsylvania; Action for Healthy Kids, Chicago, Illinois; Alliance for a Healthier Generation, New York, New York; American Academy of Pediatrics, Elk Grove Village, Illinois; American Association for Health Education, West Chester, Ohio; American Association of School Administrators, Arlington, Virginia; American Cancer Society, Atlanta, Georgia; American Dietetic Association; American Heart Association, Washington, DC; American School Health Association, Bethesda, Maryland; Consortium to Lower Obesity Among Chicago Children, Chicago, Illinois; Illinois Association of School Nurses, Wheeling, Illinois; Michigan Association of School Nurses, Troy, Michigan; National Association for Sport and Physical Education, Reston, Virginia; National Association of School Nurses, Silver Spring, Maryland; National Association of Secondary School Principals, Reston, Virginia; National Association of State Boards of Education, Arlington, Virginia; National Education Association, Washington, DC; National Food Service Management Institute, University, Mississippi; National Recreation and Parks Association, Ashburn, Virginia; National School Boards Association, Alexandria, Virginia; Prevention Institute, Oakland, California; School Nutrition Association, National Harbor, Maryland; Society for Nutrition Education, Indianapolis, Indiana; Society for Public Health Education, Washington, DC; Society of State Directors of Health, Physical Education, and Recreation, Arlington, Virginia; YMCA of the USA, Washington, DC.